Intermittent Fasting For Women

How To Improve Your Health, Increase Longevity And Lose Fat Fast Without Dieting Or Damaging Your Hormones Using The Power Of Intermittent Fasting

Rebekah Addams & Michael Russo

© Copyright 2020 by Rebekah Addams & Michael Russo- All rights reserved.

The following eBook is reproduced below with the goal of providing information that is as accurate and reliable as possible. Regardless, purchasing this eBook can be seen as consent to the fact that both the publisher and the author of this book are in no way experts on the topics discussed within and that any recommendations or suggestions that are made herein are for entertainment purposes only. Professionals should be consulted as needed prior to undertaking any of the action endorsed herein.

This declaration is deemed fair and valid by both the American Bar Association and the Committee of Publishers Association and is legally binding throughout the United States.

Furthermore, the transmission, duplication, or reproduction of any of the following work including specific information will be considered an illegal act irrespective of if it is done electronically or in print. This extends to creating a secondary or tertiary copy of the work or a recorded copy and is only allowed with the express written consent from the Publisher. All additional right reserved.

The information in the following pages is broadly considered a truthful and accurate account of facts and as such, any inattention, use, or misuse of the information in question by the reader will render any resulting actions solely under their purview. There are no scenarios in which the publisher or the original author of this work can be in any fashion deemed liable for any hardship or damages that may befall them after undertaking information described herein.

Additionally, the information in the following pages is intended only for informational purposes and should thus be thought of as universal. As befitting its nature, it is presented without assurance regarding its prolonged validity or interim quality. Trademarks that are mentioned are done without written consent and can in no way be considered an endorsement from the trademark holder.

Professional and medical disclaimer

You must not rely on the information in this book as an alternative to medical advice from your doctor or other professional healthcare provider.

If you have any specific questions regarding any medical matter, you should consult your doctor or other healthcare professional prior to beginning any nutrition and/or exercise panel.

Table of Contents

From The Author 1
Free Gift 3
Chapter 1: Obesity 4
   What Is Intermittent Fasting? 5
   Reasons to Fast 7
Chapter 2: Intermittent Fasting and FatBurning 8
   Fat Adaptation 9
   How Intermittent Fasting Improves on Fat Loss 10
Chapter 3: IF and Human Growth Hormone 12
   Fasting to Increase the Levels of the Growth Hormone 13
   Blood Levels of Human Growth Hormone 15
   Implications for the Athletes 15
   Additional Information 16
Chapter 4: IF and Insulin Sensitivity 17
   Insulin Resistance 17
   Symptoms of Insulin Resistance 18
   Insulin Resistance Tests 19
   Why Identifying Insulin Resistance Is Important 19
   Why Fasting Resolves Insulin Resistance 21
   Fasting Effectiveness Is Dependent on the Way That It Is Done 22
   Why Exercise Cannot Be a Replacement for Fasting 23
Chapter 5: Intermittent Fasting and Leptin Sensitivity 24
   The Broken Leptin System 24
   Intermittent Fasting and Leptin Resistance 26
Chapter 6: Intermittent Fasting and Brain Function. 28
   Reduction of Inflammation 28
   Autophagy 28
   Creation of More Brain Cells 29
   Boosting the Rate of Growth in the Brain 29

Burning Fat Instead of Sugar 30
Supercharging the Levels of Energy 31
What Happens to the Brain When an Animal Fasts? 31

Chapter 7: The Connection Between Intermittent Fasting and Increased Lifespan 33
Mitochondria 34
Aging and Mitochondria 35
IF and Lifespan 36
Minimalism and Lifespan 36
How Caloric Restriction Increases Lifespan 38

Chapter 8: Intermittent Fasting and Inflammation ... 39
Chronic Pain Inflammation 40
Hormone Signaling Inflammation 40
Lung Inflammation 43
Gut Inflammation 43
Intermittent Fasting and the Migrating Motor Complex 44

Chapter 9: Intermittent Fasting and Heart Health 45
Cardiac Injuries 45
Intermittent Fasting and Age-Related Hypertrophy 46
Intermittent Fasting and Coronary Heart Disease Factors .. 46

Chapter 10: Intermittent Fasting and Free Radical Damage 48

Chapter 11: Intermittent Fasting and Epilepsy 51

Chapter 12: Intermittent Fasting, Cancer, and Diabetes 53
Triggering of the Immune System in Patients 54
Efficacy in Animal Testing 55
Calorie Restriction, Fasting, and Cancer 56
How to Fast During Cancer Treatments 57
Considering Treatment Options 58
Intermittent Fasting and Diabetes 59
Timing Is Everything 62
Possible Downsides 63
Intermittent Fasting and Its Effect on Blood Sugar Control 64

Chapter 13: Understanding Food Proteins, Carbs, and Fats 68
Intermittent Fasting Meets Carb Cycling 69

 Looking out for the Plateau 71
Chapter 14: Satiety and Binge Eating 73
 Breaking Bad Eating Habits Utilizing Intermittent Fasting . 75
 False Hunger Cues 75
 Relearn the True Meaning of Hunger 76
 Making Yourself Full 76
 Principles to Feeling Satiated 77
 Feasting After the Fast 78
Chapter 15: IF For Woman 80
Chapter 16: Types of Intermittent Fasting 88
 Alternate-Days Fasting 89
 Daily Window Fasting 89
 Keto Fasting 90
 The 5:2 Diet 91
 The Warrior Diet 91
 Eat Stop Eat 92
 Leangains 93
 Fat Loss Forever 95
 Up Day Down Day 96
 My Personal Approach 97
Chapter 17 Tips for Success 99
Chapter 18: Exercise & Intermittent Fasting 102
Conclusion 105
References 107

From The Author

First of all we want to thank you and congratulate you for downloading Intermittent Fasting For Women

This book contains proven steps and strategies on how to use intermittent fasting to make losing weight effortless while still being able to eat all of your favorite comfort foods that keep satisfied through your entire journey

Even though we have both been personal trainers for over 15 years I personally (Michael) have also battled my own weight struggles. I have tried and tested many different approaches to weight loss on myself and my clients. Although many of them worked initially, they all ended up being unsustainable and thus the end result was always the same, THE WEIGHT CAME BACK ON and the yo-yo dieting continued.

I LOVE FOOD and eating 6 small meals a day every 3 hours not only took over my life but never left me full and in the end would lead to binge eating. All I wanted was to find a way that I could eat all of the foods that I loved most (not all of them overly healthy) and still lose fat and achieve a body that allowed me to be comfortable and confident in any situation.

This is a weight loss system that SIMPLY WORKS; it is easy to follow and has many other health benefits other than the weight loss which I will cover throughout this book. I go quite in depth with the health benefits that intermittent fasting can have on the body outside of weight loss but also go through many forms of Intermittent fasting including the one that I used to drop 55 pounds when I hit my heaviest after a bout of depression a few years back.

Rebekah and I have jam packed this book with as much information on what Intermittent Fasting is, how it works, how to get started and why it's the best method to achieving optimum health and a lean toned body. We truly cant wait for you to read the book, get started and achieve your own goals.

Free Gift

We would like to offer you a copy of our Intermittent Fasting Cheat Sheet that you can use for quick reference to not only get you started but also as something to refer back to whenever you need. To claim your copy just head to www.thefastingfacts.com

We would also encourage you to join our free Facebook accountability group, here you will have full access to me where we can answer any questions and help you in any way we can. This will be an extremely valuable tool to ensure your success. Please search Intermittent Fasting, Fuel the Brain, Lose the Fat and answer the 3 easy questions and we will accept you straight away.

Chapter 1: Obesity

Obesity refers to a complex disorder when a person has an excess amount of body fat. It is not just a cosmetic issue for the patient, but this also increases their apparent risk for heart disease, high blood pressure, and even diabetes. Being extremely obese is an indication that one is likely to have health issues. The great thing is that even the modest levels of weight loss may improve or even prevent the health issues linked to obesity, which, in this case, would entail changes in diet scheduling set by intermittent fasting.

Obesity is diagnosed when the body mass index (BMI) is at the level of 30 or higher. This is calculated by dividing the weight in kilograms by the height of the person. For the majority of individuals, the BMI allows a reasonable estimate of body fat. On the other hand, it is also not a direct measure of body fat. There are a few examples such as muscular athletes that have a BMI that is in the obese level category even if there is no excess body fat.

Even though the causes of body fat are generally behavioral, genetic, or hormonal influences on the levels of body weight, obesity also happens when a person takes in higher calorie levels than they are able to burn off. The body stores the excess amounts of calories as fat under the skin or around the organs. There are times when obesity may be considered to have genetic roots. For example, conditions like Prader Willy Syndrome and Cushing's Syndrome link obesity to genetic issues. These conditions are very rare though and they may only cover around 1 to 5 percent of the population. The principal causes for obesity for the majority of people out there would be:

- Unhealthy diet and eating patterns: In this case, gaining weight is inevitable if you regularly eat much more calories than are burnt off through the means of physical exercise. Many of the Western diets are too high in calories, and the patterns contain higher levels of fast food and high-calorie drinks.

- Being inactive: If a person is not active, then they do not burn as many calories. When it comes to the sluggish lifestyle, it is possible to take in more calories every day than you would use through normal daily activities and exercise.

What Is Intermittent Fasting?

Intermittent fasting (IF) is about an eating schedule where a person goes between periods of eating and fasting. The reason why this method is quite popular with people is that it does not give harsh regulations on the foods they can eat and the ones that are off-limits. Several intermittent fasting approaches may split the day patterns into a time when you fast and a time when you eat, though you need to consider people still fast when they sleep. IF could be as simplistic as trying to extend the time when you do not eat to a particular designated period. This would be possible when you do not take breakfast, eat during the afternoon, and then the last meal is done by 8 PM.

That would mean that the person is fasting for a period of 16 hours every day and that their diet is only within a period of 8 hours for every day. It is very common as a pattern of intermittent fasting, and it is dubbed as the 16-8 approach. In spite of what a lot of people think, it is quite easy to do, and the thing is that it leaves a number of people feeling better. They tend to have more energy during the later stages of the fast. There is the issue of hunger, but it is only a significant problem during the start. When the body adapts to not eating for a particular time, it starts to become easier. There is no food that is provided during the time for fasting, but there are allowances for certain drinks such as tea, coffee, and water as well as other beverages that do not have calories. A few forms of intermittent fasting give the chance for low-calorie foods during the fasted period. You are also allowed to ingest supplements provided that there are no calories within them.

The great thing with intermittent fasting is that there may be reduced levels of hunger when the person would be undergoing the diet. In the event the person is seeking to reduce their weight, it would be very beneficial as opposed to other dieting modes.
The great thing is when you skip breakfast it means you can have much more satisfying meals later in the day, something that most other diets and eating plans swear against. After a few days of doing the diet, hormones such as ghrelin allow for you to get used to the new schedule and they adjust the body so that the person does not feel hungry in the morning anymore.

Apparently, for the one doing the diet, intermittent fasting allows for something quite unique in regard to enjoying meals that are satisfying while also adhering to health benefits and losing excess weight. The lack of hunger and cravings then become one of the welcome features when it comes to intermittent fasting and add to the process of weight loss. Contrary to the main belief, the fasting phase does have a suppressive effect on the hunger levels of the individual, the hunger pains may happen sometimes but they disappear just as quickly.

The other thing is an increase in the mental focus. At the time a person is doing their fast, the body may release several stimulant hormones. You will find your focus improves and the level of productivity increases so that you feel that much more involved in everything that you are doing. It's one of my favorite parts of IF and many people see this as very apparent during the last four hours of the fast.

With fewer meals, the levels of blood sugar are then made more stable and this leads to better levels of energy and a reduction in emotional distress. The other thing is that not having to worry about meal timing because you can do it all in one period as opposed to the irritable feeling that occurs when you have to do several meals during the course of the day depending on your diet. Seriously we have family, jobs and other responsibilities, who has the time to sit down every 3 hours and eat? This might be fine for the fitness models of the world but for general people like you and me that's not always possible.

Reasons to Fast

In some cases, it is done out of necessity because there is no food available. In other cases, it is done from a religious perspective. Buddhism, Christianity, and Islam all have their forms of restriction on diet or fasting. Human beings and other animals also instinctually pass on eating food when they happen to be sick. So, there is nothing unnatural in fasting and the body is very equipped to handle extended periods without food. Everything in the body changes when people do not eat for a given time in order to allow the body to thrive during the time when there are not a lot of resources.

This has to do with hormone levels and other cellular repair processes. Many people conduct their fasting to lose weight because it is effective in burning fat. Others do it because of the metabolic health advantages as it would improve a number of risk factors. There is evidence intermittent fasting may also assist when it comes to longevity. For example, research done on rodents has illustrated intermittent fasting can extend the lifespan so long as calorie restriction is also included within this setting.

Chapter 2: Intermittent Fasting and Fat Burning

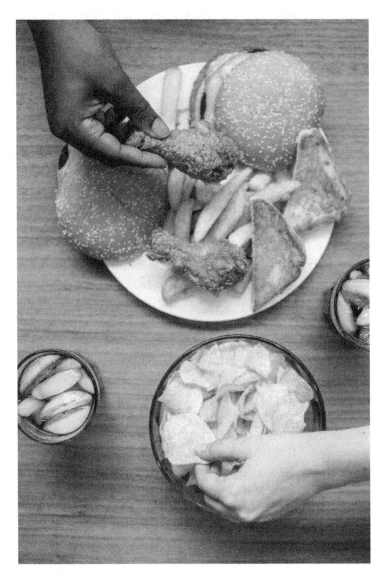

At times, weight loss can seem like a never-ending battle because people place themselves on strict diets and workout patterns that are ambitious. They are of the belief that if they punish themselves for the right amount of time, the results will be evident. This is wishful thinking though. If you have tried dieting and had to deal with constant hunger, then you know how hard it is to deal with cravings all the time. By trying to force the body to lose weight through eating less and exercising more, it would only be a short-term solution. The better approach to use is to confuse the body and minimize the level of hunger in order to take advantage of the basic ability to burn fats and lose weight in a fast manner.

The body has the ability to either use body fat or carbohydrates to generate energy. This is the flexibility the brain has for the resources at hand. On the other hand, if the person has been following a diet too rich in carbs and sugars and low in fat for the most part, then there is a great chance that their body does not follow the rules of flexibility because there is no need for it to do so. If that person goes for some time without eating and starts to feel like they are starving, then they start to become very irritable. These are some of the signs they do not have the mental flexibility that is characterized when the body turns to fat or protein in order to produce energy.

Fat Adaptation

Fat adaptation is what happens when you do have the flexibility to metabolize fats. This is what a lot of people do not have. The majority of individuals are inefficient when it comes to burning fat and so the only other option that the body has would be burning glucose and this makes them that much more dependent on carbs. They are not able to effectively sustain a state of fasting without feasting on carbs so that they are not able to reap the benefits that come with weight loss and better levels of energy. That leaves people with bad habits such as eating all the time, getting hungry constantly, not to mention developing a chain reaction for bad hormonal balances. This, in turn, affects them in different ways.

The process of becoming fat adapted happens on a cellular level as one helps their body to utilize the fats in a better manner. As this happens, the mitochondria make a number of internal changes so it becomes possible to metabolize the fat into energy. Because the majority of people are addicted to having sugar in their diet, their bodies tend to metabolize the glucose into energy as opposed to the fat. Now, the question is how long it takes for the person's body to become metabolically flexible once they start to go on the intermittent fasting regime and reduce their intake of regular sugar. The short answer is it is inconclusive but it should not be that long. This process, even if done the right way, can take different periods for different individuals. Though, if one does everything in the right manner and at the right time, then they should expect to become fat adapted within a period of 5 weeks. This would depend on how well the person keeps to their diet and maintains the fasted states. Someone that has an addiction to sugar may have a hard time trying to break the cycle.

This is not just on a mental level, but also when it comes to the physical dependency and the way the enzymes, hormones, and everything else reacts to the changes taking place. For anyone doing it to burn fats, the thing would be to trust the process and follow it so that it happens just as every other process followed through.

How Intermittent Fasting Improves on Fat Loss

It increases the amount of fat-burning hormones available in the body. Hormones are most often at the source of much of the metabolic functioning and so, when it comes to the burning of fat, this should not be different. HGH or human growth hormone, for example, is very significant in the process of burning fat. The act of fasting sets the fat burning hormone into significant production and so it makes the fat burning process go into overdrive so to speak. It would reduce insulin levels as well and this makes sure that you would burn through your body fat as opposed to storing it in the first place.

The hormones responsible for fat burning need assistance from particular enzymes to accomplish the objective. In certain scenarios, the enzymes create a particular environment that allows the fat cells to burn to create energy. The muscle tissue allows the cells to absorb fat so they can be burnt for fuel. The act of fasting increases the enzyme levels in order to optimize the burning process.

Over the short term, intermittent fasting which can be anywhere between 12 to 72 hours increases the rates of a person's metabolism and their levels of adrenaline. This would then cause the person to increase the rate of calories burnt during this time. The more calories burnt, the faster the level of weight is lost. It also means the extra energy attained from the fast would assist with getting more work done at work or even around the house. During the first fast, you may be quite surprised at how energetic and awake you are overall. The fasting time can actually turn into some of your most productive periods. In fact most of this book was written during my fasting times as that is when my concentration levels are at their peak.

Fasting tends to shift the orientation of the metabolism from burning of the blood sugar to burning the body fat. After a meal, the natural process of the metabolism is to burn the carbs first and then the fat from the food consumed. Any of the extra fat that the body is not able to consume in the first few hours after eating would be stored in the form of body fat. Now, when one fasts, the body does not have any choice but to burn the body fat which has been stored. By the end of the 24-hour fast, the body burns more fat than possible during a regular day when you take three meals.

Chapter 3: IF and Human Growth Hormone

Upon reaching the age of 30, the aging process starts, and the hormones in the body fluctuate. The process is different for everyone depending on genetics and several environmental factors, as men and women have different phases in their lives that affect the levels of their hormones. The human growth hormone is produced by the pituitary gland and contributes to the growth and development in adolescents. The deficiency of human growth hormone in adult means higher body fat and reduced muscle mass and bone density. Once it is availed from the pituitary gland, the human growth hormone only lasts a short time in the blood. From there, it finds its way to the liver where it is metabolized and initiated into growth factors.

That would be the same, which is linked to high levels of insulin that leads to several health issues. However, the brief instance of the growth factors from human growth hormone lasts only a few minutes. All of the hormones are secreted naturally and done so in brief bursts in order to prevent the initiation of some resistance which is what happens when the body gets used to high levels of the hormone in the bloodstream without acting proportionately to their secretion. The first discoveries of human growth hormone came from experiments on cadavers done in the 50s though it was synthesized in a lab environment during the 80s. After that, it became very popular as a performance enhancing supplement. The normal levels of the hormone in a person tend to reach a peak during the time of puberty as would be expected, and they decrease gradually afterward. Growth hormone tends to be produced when a person is sleeping and is one of the counter-regulatory hormones that are produced naturally. Both cortisol and HGH increases the level of glucose in the bloodstream by breaking down the glycogen in order that it counters the effects that are rendered by insulin. Insulin reduces the amount of blood glucose levels while HGH increases blood glucose.

These hormones are usually secreted in pulses before a person wakes up. This would be deemed normal and it is supposed to get the body ready for the day through pushing the glucose out of storage and into the bloodstream where it is then available for energy creation. When someone says that a person needs to eat their breakfast in order for them to have the right energy levels for the day, this is very incorrect. The body has already provided enough resources for this to happen so there is no need to do cereals or a heavy breakfast in order to get the fuel needed for the day. This is why hunger happens to be its lowest during the early morning even if someone has not eaten during the night unless the body has already been conditioned to consume food during this time, which is what happens with most people.

Fasting to Increase the Levels of the Growth Hormone

In 1982, Kerndt produced a study that was of a single patient and they went through a 40-day fast for religious needs. The glucose levels decreased, from a level of 96, it dropped to a level of 56. The insulin went much lower and stabilized. The concern was the HGH though. According to the study taken, it started at a level of 0.74 typically and would peak at 9.86. That would mean a 1,250% increase in the level of the growth hormone. Even a fast for five days gives a significant increase in the growth hormone.

This is all according to research done on the subject. The question then goes to the potential side effects of the increased growth hormone from fasting. There might be an increased level of blood sugar for someone but there is hardly a risk for the potential of debilitating lifestyle diseases such as cancer and diabetes.

Fasting is seen as one of the great stimulating factors for HGH secretion. During the time of fasting, there happens to be a spike during the morning period, but there is usually some secretion going on during the day as well. The HGH is crucial after all to maintain and develop muscle fiber and bone density. Though, some of the main issues that come with fasting include the decreased levels of muscle mass. There are some that say fasting a single day would even cause a loss of about ¼ of a pound of muscle. In fact, the opposite is said to happen according to verified research. In comparing the caloric reduction diets to fasting, the fasting was much better at the preservation of lean mass.

Say that somebody is living during the prehistoric Paleolithic era. During the summer when there's an abundance of food, the community would engage in a lot of feasting and then store some of that as fat within the body. During the time of winter, there would be nothing to eat. The question is whether the body would metabolize the muscle but preserve the stored fat. In this case, the body would start to burn the stored fat instead of the precious muscle fiber. It is true though, that some protein is catabolized for the purposes of gluconeogenesis, though the increase in HGH maintains lean mass during the time of fasting.

The increases in human growth hormone when a person is fasting assist in preserving the muscle tissue and the stores of glycogen while using the fat stores instead. This breakdown of the fat in a process known as lipolysis releases glycerol and other fatty acids, which would be metabolized for the creation of energy. Madelon Buijs, who is a researcher at the Leiden University Medical Center in the Netherlands, claims the increases in HGH rise noticeably during the first 13 hours of beginning a fast which would mean an increased breakdown of fats during the first half of the day of the fast.

Blood Levels of Human Growth Hormone

In the cases of a lack of human growth hormone when fasting, loss of protein from the muscles increases by 50 percent. Though, fasting and exercise during the fast may lend to an increase in the levels of growth hormone. They are also subject to a lot of variation taking place during the day because the pituitary gland releases the hormone in particular bursts. The random evaluation of the levels of human growth hormone as opposed to monitoring it over a period of time is not necessarily useful as well. Though, levels during the morning would be much higher than the ones that are recorded during the course of the day.

Implications for the Athletes

This has significant ramifications for the athletes as it is known as training during the fasting phase. The increase of adrenaline from the fasting is going to increase motivation so that the person will train harder. Similarly, the increased levels of HGH as stimulated by the intermittent fasting will result in a toning effect and an increase in muscle mass that will help in making recovery from the workout sessions that much easier. That would be a significant advantage for the athletes, especially in the endurance department. There is also a lot of new attention that is being given to this approach to muscle treatment and exercise. It is not happenstance that many of the early proponents in training during the fasting state are bodybuilders. This is because it is a sport that requires a lot of high-intensity training and very low levels of body fat.

There is even a book written by bodybuilder Brad Pilon known as 'Eat, Stop, Eat' which popularized the lean gains approach to fasting. For those individuals who believed fasting would increase the levels of fatigue and make you tired or it would not be possible to exercise during fasting, that is a wrong mentality.

Fasting in itself does not cause you to burn muscle fiber significantly. There is no typical approach, meaning you have to shrivel up into a skeleton in order to get effective results from the fasted state. The difference with those scenarios is the individuals illustrated did not receive any form of nourishment during their fasts and could even go weeks without sufficient water and food between days. At that level, you would be punishing your body rather than taming it and the situations are due to lack rather than active choice because no one can hold out that long.

As such, fasting when done right has good potential in creating anti-aging properties that are brought about by human growth hormone without the potential problems created by excess HGH such as increased blood pressure and prostate cancer. For the ones that are interested in competing at an elite or athletic level, then the benefits would be much better for them.

Additional Information

The testing that comes with HGH is not particularly routine. At times, it is done in order to help diagnose the pituitary issues that can at times lead to conditions like gigantism or stunted growth. Even though HGH therapy is approved when it comes to treating those children that have stunted growth, it has also attracted a lot of attention because of the effects that it has been deemed to have on muscle and fat tissues. Synthetic HGH is available for purchase though not a lot is known about the long-term safety it has on the subject.

Chapter 4: IF and Insulin Sensitivity

When you eat and the body proceeds to break down the food, sugars from the material consumed are transported to the cells. This is the glucose that is metabolized by the mitochondria in order to create energy for the cells and tissues to function, as they should. Insulin, the hormone that informs the cells they need to accept the glucose as it is delivered. When the body attains the signal that consumption has taken place, cells known as beta cells in the pancreas release the insulin hormone. Insulin tells the cells in the body to absorb the glucose being broken down from the carbs or fat, or in rare cases, protein. When a person does not have insulin, as in the case of a diabetic, then the cells do not allow glucose in; hence, it stays within the bloodstream. Once the body gets the sense that glucose has been around within the bloodstream for a period of time, then it stores it as fat for later use because it believes that the cells are not in need of it.

Insulin Resistance

When insulin issues a signal to the cells that the fuel is on the way, the cells then make a response through getting the glucose from the bloodstream. Each of the cells gets the energy needed to perform their functions which translates to adequate body processes. Though, there are times when the communication gets thrown off. Insulin resistance is what happens hypothetically when the body is notified by the insulin but there is no significant response to it. The insulin may issue a sign that fuel is coming to the cells so they need to be ready but the cells may not open up to absorb the glucose. In this case, the sugar may continue to stay within the bloodstream, and after a bit of time, the body then packs it as extra fat.

When the cells do not accept the sugar in order to convert it into energy, the result is the body detects that something is wrong and in response sends more insulin through the pancreas to ascertain what is wrong as if trying to fix the problem by delivering a higher dose. Sometimes, a little more insulin may be what the cells need in order to respond and in turn accept the glucose so that it can be turned into fat. The insulin resistance is what happens when the cells continue to ignore the insulin signals for various reasons. Now, this conversely results in overworking the pancreas, as it is not aware why the body is not converting the sugar into glucose at the appropriate rate yet it is funneling insulin into the system. When the pancreas gets fatigued because of the overproduction rates, then there is a possibility it can fail, leading to insulin deficiency and prediabetes.

Symptoms of Insulin Resistance

Most people happen to be insulin resistant and not aware of it. They may go for years or even their entire lives without having the energy they could have. A lot of the time, the insulin resistance may not be at the level where it causes any symptoms at all and the ones that do show up can be attributed to a host of other conditions that are non-related. Some of those things that could be attributed to insulin resistance would include the following:

- Elevated levels of blood sugar due to fasting
- Acne
- Fatty liver disease   ☐ Sugar cravings
- High blood pressure
- Fluid retention
- Trouble concentrating
- Scalp hair loss
- Skin tags

Now, all of these symptoms on their own are relatively mild or they could be considered as signs of other underlying issues, which is why insulin resistance is a bit hard to catch right off the bat.

Insulin Resistance Tests

Functional medicine and conventional medical personal doctors treat the numbers in a different manner. Usually, the conventional doctors will consider broader ranges as the norm even when there are symptoms. Only when one is out of range would they treat it and this is centered on prescriptions that have less attention to lifestyle and dieting. Functional medicine, on the other hand, works in a different manner. The first thing is that conventional laboratories consider middle proportions of the people tested as the normal. That is to say, the numbers change according to the ones that have been tested. The question is if you want someone to decide if the numbers are okay compared to a human or when they are set against a group of individuals in one of the sickest developed nations in the world.

The other thing is conventional medical doctors treat the prescriptions and symptoms as puzzle pieces they utilize in order for them to arrive at a particular diagnosis. Laboratory testing is not necessarily the main determinant in this scenario. The third thing to consider would be treatment involving things such as diet and changes in lifestyle and prescriptions when completely significant. Now, there are blood tests that will be needed in order to determine the insulin sensitivity and the ranges in conventional medicine that functional practitioners use when compared to the conventional medical professionals.

Why Identifying Insulin Resistance Is Important

There are two types of diabetes. These would be type 1, also referred to as an insulin-dependent mode of diabetes and type 2 diabetes. This is related to the lifestyle of the individual. Type 2 usually accounts for 90 to 95 percent of the cases of diabetes and its cases started to become quite significant during the time of the 80s when obesity was yet to be one of the more significant trends. The underlying problem that concerns type 2 diabetes would be the insulin resistance that comes along with it. The body could be producing a large amount of insulin in order to force that glucose into the cells. Hence, if there is a need for the body to produce up to four times the normal amount to shove the glucose into the cells, then there is a problem which is not easily detectable if you were only to measure the levels of the blood glucose.

Through the utilization of the Kraft assay, which considers how much the insulin is increasing within the bloodstream, it becomes possible to detect the insulin resistance when it is at an earlier stage. This would be significant considering there are things that can be done about reversing the process. Insulin resistance that ends in mitochondrial issues is one of the main factors behind Alzheimer's, cancer, and other diseases that degenerate the body.

Why Fasting Resolves Insulin Resistance

Fasting has been used for thousands of years in order to keep people fit. Once insulin resistance becomes evident in what it is, then it is possible to understand why something simple like abstaining from food for a period of time can be strong as a means for intervention. Contrary to infectious diseases, it is not possible to treat metabolic diseases with the use of pills because diseases like diabetes are predicated on the main diet and lifestyle.

The best means for one to counter the levels of insulin resistance is through fasting. According to Jason Fung, intermittent fasting reduces the levels of insulin, which then alters the demand for insulin but in a good way. If one is to become quite insulin resistant, then the levels of insulin would be on a high all of the time. The body seems to be always trying to shove the energy into the fat cells and a person then feels cold and really bad. That is the main resistance which is dependent on two things. It is not just the high levels but also the persistence that comes with these levels. As concerns the effects of intermittent fasting on insulin sensitivity, researchers have arrived at significant results utilizing one study where it worked at a better rate than continuous energy restriction.

Fasting Effectiveness Is Dependent on the Way That It Is Done

Time-restricted feeding and intermittent fasting are advantageous as they include periods of food avoidance. The evidence on its particular efficacy, when it comes to improving insulin sensitivity, is valid even though it is dependent on the way that it is done. Two research studies considered the concept by having their subjects eat normally one day and they would fast on the second day. This schedule was repeated seven times over a time of two weeks and there were results found where one reported an improvement in the insulin sensitivity while the other study did not observe any such benefit. In an alternative approach, people were confined to eating during a particular window every day. In this case, there were significant improvements in the levels of insulin sensitivity.

A distinction though has to be made between thoughtful restriction of food and starvation. Though fasting and time restricted eating relates as a deliberate restriction of the food on a daily basis or for longer, each of these is a scheme that entails eating fully for a period with deliberate restrictions done for only particular periods. These would be a part of each day supposedly or every now and then. Ideally speaking, there is no calorie counting with either strategy, as it would just be avoiding consuming at particular times and eating normally to the point of satisfaction.

It may seem a bit fussy but there is a fine line between eating to keep within the levels of insulin low as opposed to just starving the body. When taken to the absolute extreme, it is possible that fasting may result in much more harm to the system than good. There is no definite time past which fasting becomes counterproductive so a lot is dependent on the constitution of the individual that is fasting and their definitions for fasting along with how they are compensating for not consuming some of the essential nutrients.

There is research into prolonged durations of fasting which has found potentially hazardous consequences after the fasting ends and this is known as 're-feeding syndrome'. If it is not conducted in the right manner, prolonged fasting then turns into starvation and that would make the body become insulin resistant which is ironic.

Why Exercise Cannot Be a Replacement for Fasting

In order to avoid adding sugar to the bloodstream, it is crucial for a people to adopt a cyclical low carb and high-fat type of diet. In order to burn off the glucose that is already within the system, intermittent fasting comes in handy. Though, exercise does not represent a solution for the insulin resistance and subsequent diabetes. The reason for this is you do not only have insulin resistance within the muscle fiber but also in the tissues and other organs and systems in the body. This is a body problem rather than a regional issue and so to eliminate the excess glucose that is in the tissues, the best way to go about it would be to temporarily starve the cells so they would have to burn off the glucose. Clearly, it is also important for people to exercise as much as they can, but this is only going to result in burning the glycogen that is in the muscle fibers. It is not going to be of much help to the fat around the liver or the visceral fat around other organs in the body. Apparently, fasting disposes of all the excess nutrients. That is why historically, people denoted it as a form of cleansing or a detox because that is exactly what is going on.

Chapter 5: Intermittent Fasting and Leptin Sensitivity

Leptin is a hormone that is released by fat cells in adipose tissue. It is regulated through evaluation of the fat mass within the body. A drop, therefore, in the level of leptin would significantly affect the other hormones negatively. Low levels of leptin increase hunger, which means decreasing the rates of metabolism. That implies lean or thin people tend to have low leptin levels, but those who are fat have much higher leptin levels. Leptin resistance is a high probability in those who have more fat. This is due to the periodically increased leptin that is like insulin resistance in the sense that the resistance comes from periodically elevated insulin.

The theory concerning body weight regulation links leptin to mass using a genetic argument. Naturally, thin people tend to have a low level of body fat set because they are leptin sensitive leading to a low body fat percentage. They operate in the right manner at these low levels of leptin, but many people are not that lucky.

The Broken Leptin System

Leptin may communicate on the level of fat within the system to balance the energy needs. Because it is created by fat cells, there is a direct correlation to the quantity. A higher amount of fat means more levels of leptin. When the fat store is full, the satisfaction signal is sent, and this prevents you from eating more.

Now, when there are low stores of fat, a signal is also sent telling the body that it is starving and it needs to increase consumption. This is a negative feedback thing as when there are fat stores, the need to consume calories is not there. When people are overweight, they tend to have a large number of cells which means a lot of leptin.

The increased creation of leptin along with insulin is common in obesity situations and causes resistance within the brain. The brain loses sensitivity to signals provided by leptin illustrating the level of the fat stores. That effectively means it tampers with the satiety signals. Leptin resistance from the high levels of leptin is a key psychological issue behind obesity. However, loss of weight and fat cells may trigger the need for consuming a higher level of calories. During the loss of leptin and the fat cells, there is not an automatic reset on the brain.

Reducing the circulation of leptin may trigger a starvation signal from the brain and that means an increased level of appetite. Losing weight may also not be the only cause for a deficiency of leptin. There are particular genetic defects that contribute to low levels of leptin. The approximation is 3 percent of people have receptor malfunctions which contribute to their obesity. In America, that entails an estimated 2,300,000. Inflammation within the hypothalamus in the brain has also been shown to cause some form of leptin resistance.

Overall, it is a difficult phenomenon to treat and this is mostly due to the fact that the body seems to want to hold on to whichever body fat is available. It has now become verifiable that the major role of the hormone is defending against the reductions of body fat, which would lead to threats to survival and future reproduction. It may seem a bit counterproductive because that would increase the risk of developing obesity within people. Though it does make sense considering it would have worked well for people of the Paleolithic era who alternated between fasting and feasting so they were at a lower risk of obesity as compared to modern civilization.

Intermittent Fasting and Leptin Resistance

Several studies illustrated neutral effects on average leptin levels during an intermittent fast. However, the fasting period could result in a reduction of the leptin though this would be compensated through a boost during re-feeding. When paired with the usual meal schedule, intermittent fasting infuses patterns of peak and valley as concerns leptin synthesis. Leptin secrets are then entrained to the meal patterns and shifts of meal timing, which could lead to a shift in the leptin rhythm. It would seem there are differences on this matter as females, in particular, may illustrate increases in their average leptin during fasted periods. It even occurs when there is zero weight gain.

Intermittent fasting has also seen to be able to reduce the levels of hormones that stimulate hunger. This is illustrated through the increased leptin levels even though there does not seem to be a particular link between the two in this scenario. There are similar effects that have been found to happen in men though. That would be to say that fat loss occurred without clear reductions in leptin levels, though it should be noted that these were lean athletes. So intermittent fasting can be of benefit when it comes to dieting within the single digit range because of the effect the process has on fat mobilizing hormones like epinephrine and norepinephrine. When you are in the single digit body fat range, then there is a high chance of having low levels of leptin. Part of the downstream effects of the hormone concerns both norepinephrine and epinephrine. Low levels of leptin lead to reduced or impaired production of both the hormones.

This is part of the reason the leptin would manipulate metabolism rates. However, it could be that hormones may increase regardless during the fasted period. Therefore, leptin is not able to exert itself as normal over the system hormones. In such a case, an increase in their levels in the system would not be medicated through leptin utilization that allows for things like fat mobilization during the fasting period.

Chapter 6: Intermittent Fasting and Brain Function

Fasting has its advantages in relation to a range of the different functions of the brain. When it comes to the cellular cleansing process, one of the advantages includes autophagy activation. Both humans and mammals respond in the same manner when they are deprived of calories. The size of their organs can shrink significantly.

Reduction of Inflammation

Intermittent fasting has been illustrated to significantly reduce the levels of inflammation within people. An excessive amount of inflammation would be the reason behind several chronic diseases that we are hearing more and more about in this current day and age such as obesity, dementia, and Alzheimer's.

Autophagy

As discussed earlier, this is a very significant topic when it comes to intermittent fasting and the advantages it gives to brain function. Autophagy is what happens when the body destroys the old or the damaged cells. You should think of it like cleaning the rust and allowing it to cleanse. If the damaged or the old cells remain within the body, they tend to create an inflammation situation. Therefore, intermittent fasting stimulates more autophagy within the brain which basically means it assists the brain to clean itself and reduce the inflammation. Through activating the process, a person is then able to reduce inflammation and optimize on the brain functions while slowing down the aging process. A lot of research has been done which proves that fasting promotes the act of autophagy within the brain. Thus, it is able to increase the cognitive functions by improving the brain structure and reducing the inflammations as they happen which denature the brain.

- Ketones: Even though this is an article on intermittent fasting, this has to be mentioned as it has to do with the connection between fasting and brain activity. When you are fasting, the body uses up the sugar stores and as a result has to turn to fat for the fuel. When the fat breaks down, ketones are released, and they are used for energy for the body and brain activities. One of the most significant ketones strengthens the part of the immune system that handles the regulating of inflammatory disorders such as Alzheimer's and arthritis.

Creation of More Brain Cells

This may seem like the opposite of what intermittent fasting would do for the brain as everywhere else it encourages the burning up of fat stores in order to create energy and run the body in a more optimal manner. According to research from John Hopkins University, it seems that fasting has been shown to be behind the neurological development in the brain. This is the initiation and development of new brain cells and tissues. In turn, higher rates of this cell and tissue development within the brain have been linked to increased brain performance, mood and even focus. One study, for example, illustrated that intermittent fasting particularly stimulated the production of new brain cells.

Boosting the Rate of Growth in the Brain

Apparently, fasting does not only increase the rate of neurological development, as it also boosts the production of a protein that is referred to as BDNF. It stimulates accelerated growth within the brain. BDNF has been illustrated to play a role when it comes to neurogenesis and that allows the brain to grow and adapt adequately. It makes the brain better equipt in adapting to stress and agreeable to changes within the environment. At the time BDNF is released, there are new connections that form in the brain, and they result in the attraction of new dendrites from the nerve cells so they can connect to others. As the synapses fire, they form new connections and networks. This is the way thought processes and memory are formed and consolidated. The fast form of learning is necessary when it comes to emergency situations where fight or flight could be the only means of coping. So the benefits of BDNF include that it allows for the survival of the current neurons. They also encourage such things like differentiation and the growth of the new neurons and synapses through the means of neurogenesis. BDNF also contributes to learning, memory, and thought. On the other hand, BDNF deficiencies have been linked to several developmental disorders along with depression.

Now, diets high in carbs or sugar tend to reduce the levels of BDNF which makes sense because intermittent fasting allows one to burn off their glucose levels thereby reducing the blood sugar.

Burning Fat Instead of Sugar

This harks to the creation of energy through the means of fat stores rather than carbs and is claimed to be the better and cleaner source of energy among the two. Apparently, fat, apart from producing more energy per gram also creates less free radicals that may cause inflammation. When the mitochondria use ketones from fat or carbs to create energy, there are free radicals that are initiated, and this is the waste. The free radicals cause oxidative stresses to the body and they are claimed to be the cause for a number of neuro-linked diseases currently. So it would seem that reducing the levels of free radicals would coincide with reducing the blood sugar levels so that the body instead turns to the fat stores.

Supercharging the Levels of Energy

Intermittent fasting has been illustrated to be able to boost the mitochondrial biogenesis which is the production of mitochondria, the battery of the cells. Every cell has hundreds of mitochondria and their tasks are to issue the right energy levels for the cell to carry out its activities. They take the food that is consumed and broken down and turn it into energy within the cells so they can go about their functions. Within the brain, the mitochondria allow for synapse firing and other processes that further cognitive functioning. As such, intermittent fasting allows for the creation of more batteries within the brain so that it can become more efficient and longer lasting supposedly.

What Happens to the Brain When an Animal Fasts?

When an animal such as a wolf or a cougar has not killed any prey for a few weeks, during that time they are mostly running on ketones as their glucose stores have been burned out. As such, it is important that their brain and body are able to process well during the fasted state as they look for more prey and that is what has been found through experimentation with lab animals. The brain and the body apparently perform much better during the period of fasting. In the case of the brain, learning, memory and cognitive function and alertness all increase through fasting. In the body, it has been concluded that mice maintained better physical performance when they were placed on an intermittent fasting schedule.

In animals within the lab, fasting and exercise have been found to provide stimulation for the production of proteins within nerve cells known as brain-derived neurodevelopmental factors which have been covered as BDNF. That would mean that the same benefits derived from BDNF within people theoretically have been proven in animals. So, neurons tend to be in a resource conservation mode for stress resistance during fasting. Through extrapolation, when the animal and human eat after fasting, the neurons then go to a process of growth mode where they make a lot of proteins and they form new synapses.

Chapter 7: The Connection Between Intermittent Fasting and Increased Lifespan

Intermittent fasting has become all the rage these days — thanks to its many benefits. People have found different variations to make intermittent fasting suited for them, and this has resulted in positive outcomes. Research has proven that this type of fasting has had a positive impact on those who participate. However, we still do not have enough understanding of the underlying biological mechanism at play. One of these positive outcomes is an increased lifespan. There is much that has been said about this outcome, and a lot of controversies have surrounded the topic. Many participate in intermittent fasting for the dietary and health benefits. Rarely will a person commit to it because they believe it will increase their lifespan, as they don't believe it. Up until recently, there was no scientific evidence to back up this claim. However, a study conducted at Harvard T.H. Chan School of Public Health showed that intermittent fasting can actually increase your lifespan. So, how exactly does intermittent fasting increase your lifespan?

There are some promising animal studies that have shown that dietary restriction including the restriction of calories and intermittent fasting can delay the process of aging and extend a healthy lifespan in yeast, mice, and monkeys. The study that was published in Cell Metabolism explores the basic biology of the cells' decreasing ability to process energy as time goes by. It also sheds light on how interventions such as fasting will promote healthy aging and a healthy lifespan. The study was keen on mitochondria because it is the powerhouse of all cells.

Mitochondria are the structures in cells that produce energy. They exist in networks that change in shape dynamically according to the demand of energy in the cells. The ability of the mitochondria to keep changing in shape keeps on declining as a person ages. The impact of this on the metabolism and cell function of the person was found to be unclear. Finally, the study concluded that there is a link between the change in shape of the mitochondria networks and an increased lifespan.

The molar mechanism of intermittent fasting and other forms of dietary restriction involves the removal or improvement of the function of the cells that have been damaged or the senescent cells that have been noted by the body and have been prevented from dividing. The damaged cells have mitochondria that cannot change in shape and thus their 'productivity' is less than the rest are. Unfortunately, it is quite difficult to study aging and senescence cell biomarkers in human beings. This is because most people cannot and will not participate in any long-term intervention studies; therefore, data from human studies are very rare and this applies to studies involving IF (intermittent fasting) and calorie restriction. Because humans are difficult to study, the scientists at Harvard T.H. Chan School of Public Health used C. elegans (popularly known as nematode worms) to conduct their research.

Nematode worms only live for two weeks, which makes them perfect for studying aging in real time in the laboratories. In order to understand the study, we must first take a brief look at how the mitochondria function in the body in relation to aging and lifespan.

Mitochondria

The mitochondria are small. They measure between 0.75 and 3 micrometers, and so they cannot be viewed under a microscope unless they are stained. One main characteristic of Mitochondria is that they are divided into different regions that carry out different roles in the body. For example, there are the cristae, which are the folds of the inner membrane. They increase their surface area of the inner membrane for chemical reactions to occur at a higher rate. Another part of the mitochondria is the matrix. It is the gap that is inside the inner membrane. It contains hundreds of enzymes that are necessary for the production of ATP which is for energy creation.

Adenosine Triphosphate or ATP is the main carrier of energy in all living organisms. Every organism that is considered to be 'alive' is known to metabolize food in order to collect and store energy in the form of ATP. When the body requires energy, the ATP is broken down through hydrolysis; here, the high-energy bond is broken down and a phosphoric group is extracted. The energy that is produced through this breaking down is used for the proper functioning of various cellular processes. ATP is always being formed in the body because it is important for biological functions. Without the ATP, cells would not be able to transfer energy from one part of the body to the other which would prevent growth and reproduction.

ATP is present in all living things and active microbial cells, so it is an accurate indicator of the microbiological content that is in fluids or deposits. A great example of this is the process by which the tail of a firefly lights up. The process is a chemical reaction that occurs between luciferase and ATP. Through the measuring of ATP release from dead cells, cause and effect relationships can be identified which in turn can help you solve any microbiological changes.

Aging and Mitochondria

Another characteristic of mitochondria is that they have their own genetic material that is close to the form of DNA molecules. According to one theory proposed over half a century ago, aging of cells is linked to the constant delivery of reactive oxygen species or ROS (whose function is to regulate physiological processes) inside mitochondria through the course of life. ROS then damages the mitochondrial DNA because it is not protected by repairing enzymes like DNA. The damage of the mitochondrial DNA, in turn, leads to a deficiency of electron transport enzymes and the proper generation of ROS. This results in a sudden drop in the energy that is produced.

Another theory that has linked aging to mitochondria is the theory of mitochondria permeability. The theory implies that the level of permeability of the inner mitochondrial membrane experiences a sudden increase. Research has shown that this opening occurs because of a non-specific pore.

IF and Lifespan

Normally, mitochondrial networks inside of cells alternate between two states; fragmented and fused states. The researchers restricted the diet of the worms to discover that the mitochondrial networks remained to be youthful. This occurred through the genetic manipulation of an energy-sensing protein that is scientifically known an AMPK, which stands for an activated protein kinase. Therefore, we can confirm that when you block the mitochondria in just one state, this in turn blocks the effects of dietary restriction and fasting on longevity. The study is still quite new and though there has been some scientific foundation on the relationship between IF and an increased lifespan, studies are still being conducted to better understand the underlying biology on this phenomenon.

Minimalism and Lifespan

Researchers have clearly been considering the link between the quality of a person's life and the diet they take since the 70s when doctors noticed long-term benefits that came with extreme fasting on people that were considering weight loss seriously. According to a case in 1973, a 27-year-old man that had a weight of more than 450 pounds lost an excess of 270 pounds after placing a lot of caloric restrictions and maintained the level of his weight throughout the next few years after that. Studies have apparently gone beyond the consideration of weight and has transcended into the connection of a healthier food based diet and an increase in lifespan. Researchers in Japan also came to the realization that if people ate particular foods such as fish, fruits, and meat, then they would have the tendency of a lower rate of mortality. Closer adherence as well to the Japanese style of diet was linked with a lower overall risk level of cardiovascular disease especially when it came to cerebrovascular disease in the older people.

Now, fasting has been connected to a higher chance of curing cancer through better exposure of the cancer cells to the immune system. However, there is not a lot of data which supports the claim that people in nations which fast the most also tend to live the longest life considering that life expectancy and fasting are influenced through a number of factors.

When considered from a religious perspective, fasting is done differently around the world as dependent on the cultural and religious setting as Ramadan, for example, this is a celebration that happens between May and June.

Now, according to minimalism culture and relevant studies that were done on fasting within the region, it has been found that Singapore, Korea, and Japan all top the list for life expectancy.
The most recent data from the world health organization places Japan as the one with the longest life expectancy at 83.7 years while Singapore is third at 83.1. On the other hand, data also links low life expectancy with a lot of meat and poultry consumption, though, according to the global data as concerns the meat consumption, Japan is within the middle area.

How Caloric Restriction Increases Lifespan

Most of the other genetic pathways that have been discussed have also been associated with energy efficiency and the deprivation of nutrients. When the body faces a shortage of energy whether through fasting or starvation, then it is going to promote the fusion of mitochondria. That would then lower the energetic demands considering the organelles within the cells happen to be in better connection. This will also allow the person to be able to recycle some of the worn-out cell components and convert them back into energy via autophagy. Microphagy refers to a deeper layer considering the mitochondrial fission-fusion cycle. The energy restriction would also up-regulate the other genes increasing energy efficiency through improvement of the fat oxidation and the insulin sensitivity. During the states of fasting and the depletion of the calories, the mitochondria increase the level of their functioning. At a tissue level, this is advantageous for improving the aging process and would be felt over the long term by optimizing body functions leading to longer life apart from the obvious health advantages given.

Chapter 8: Intermittent Fasting and Inflammation

One of the main phenomena of high-fat diets and their induced obesity would be the development of inflammation, and this is prevalent in white adipose tissue. Inflammation (which will be covered in this chapter) will cover other areas in the body where it can occur due to poor dieting and how intermittent fasting can help relieve the situation.

As reviewed, it has been found that inflammation can mediate sickness symptoms and memory deficits, thereby making them worse so we need to consider what fasting does to these effects.

Inflammation is not always a good or bad kind of response within the body. It happens when the body is trying to heal itself. However, when the inflammation lasts for long periods of time, there are negative health effects that can happen. Chronic inflammation is involved in many of the present chronic conditions such as gastrointestinal diseases like Crohn's disease, obesity, asthma, and cancer. You also need to consider the fact that inflammation is a major cause of musculoskeletal disorders from short-term back pain to osteoporosis and arthritis. There are recent studies that have since drawn a positive relation between fasting and chronic instances of inflammation.

Leukotriene B4 has a significant role to play when it comes to several cellular processes when it comes to inflammation such as enzyme release, oxidative metabolism and the stimulation of neutrophil migration, and aggregation. It is a known fact that the changing of the intake of a persons lipids changes the phospholipid and fatty acid composition of the cell membranes.

Chronic Pain Inflammation

Intermittent fasting has been found to be behind something known as neuroplasticity or the ability of the brain to form and reorganize the connections in response to new information. The researchers are currently studying this and the role that it plays in the management of chronic pain. There are times when someone can feel chronic pain on their leg or another part of their body that isn't attributed to anything medical. Instead, it is said to be a psychological issue. The pain sensations coming from the muscles, bones, joints or the skin send messages to the brain and that is how these sensations are perceived by the brain in order to make the person writhe in agony. If the person suffers from chronic pain, one thing to notice is the intensity of their pain can change with their mood, the perception of their past experiences, or how bad they believe the condition is. As such, neuroplasticity brought on by intermittent fasting allows for better connections between the neurons, which means a clearer cognitive function and perceptions of pain. At the very least, stabilizing of mood and elimination of brain fog is going to at least ease situations of phantom pain and chronic pain inflammation.

Hormone Signalling Inflammation

Intermittent fasting decreases such things as leptin and insulin resistance is a hormonal issue affecting a significant percentage of the population. It also increases the production of enzymes deemed to be beneficial which increase the ability of the body to adapt to stress and fight chronic diseases such as diabetes. Calorie restriction through intermittent fasting affects the levels of energy and oxygen radical metabolism and cellular response systems in ways that would protect neurons against environmental and genetic factors. There are several interactive pathways and molecular mechanisms by which calorie restriction and intermittent fasting benefit neurons including the ones that involve insulin such as signaling, sirtuins, peroxisome proliferator-activated receptors, and FoxO transcription factors. These are some of the pathways that stimulate the production of neurodevelopment factors and antioxidant enzymes that assist the cells to cope with stress and resist disease.

A better understanding of the effects of calorie restrictions and intermittent fasting on the nervous system would lead to better approaches concerning the prevention and treatment of these disorders.

Lung Inflammation

There have been studies which showed that fasting, when done every other day, has been illustrated to decrease the symptoms related to asthma and the markers of oxidative stress. It would be interesting to note that obesity is a risk element for asthma so fasting can improve symptoms related to the inflammation that comes with these conditions. Though the trouble is several patients have never thought to adhere to low-calorie type diets and the effects of dietary restrictions on the disease has not been researched well.

Gut Inflammation

Fasting reduces the oxidative stress via the genes. This is damage that happens to the cells from exposure to toxic materials. The lipids, proteins, and DNA are affected, and they then change the functions of the cells so that they become malignant. This process is what antioxidants prevent so it is important for you to activate them. As a result, the development of irritable bowel syndrome is connected to increased levels of the oxidative enzymes and reduced activity of the antioxidant enzymes. This is what may cause progressive damage to the cells and hold back their function.

The progressive damage done to one organ in the digestive system can throw the entire process out of order, which then results in conditions such as irritable bowel syndrome. Fasting could be one of the most powerful interventions for a leaky gut and irritable bowel syndrome because of the reduction in the oxidative stress; exposure to toxicity is minimized, and the inflammation is subdued, therefore the cells of the body could have room in order for them to regenerate.

Intermittent Fasting and the Migrating Motor Complex

At the heart of several of the symptoms, related to irritable bowel syndrome would be the bacteria inside the gut. There are such things like dysbiosis or microbial imbalance as well as small intestinal bacterial overgrowth. This is to mean that the microbial community in the gut is not in order, which then causes a leaky gut. The interesting thing is fasting could assist with shaping the composition of the gut microbiome which is controlled through the MMC. The MMC refers to a mechanism which regulates the small intestinal contractions and the stomach in a cyclical pattern over the course of 2 hours. The basic function is to perform housecleaning throughout the tract which in turn sweeps the bacteria and undigested food so they can be eliminated through egestion.

The MMC is directed through a number of neuro-hormonal signals that are a response to either consumption or the feeding of the person and these hormones can be motilin, serotonin, somatostatin, and ghrelin. The activity of MMC peaks between different meals when there is no food. The presence of food is what interrupts the MMC and thus steers the hormonal activities back to assimilation and breaking down of the nutrients. When the MMC is provided with the time and space so that it can operate, it becomes harder for the food and bacteria to still be there. This is the reason as to why fasting may be viable as antiSIBO measures.

The patients that have SIBO also have absent or disrupted patterns concerning MMC patterns. The patients that went through irritable bowel syndrome had shorter durations for motor activity when compared to the healthier counterparts. When and how you decide eating may induce a number of changes in the gut microbiome and this then contributes to the diversity that is related to the gut microbes. This presents a process by which the bacteria affect metabolism, immunity, as well as digestion. There is only one study which has investigated the impacts on things such as fasting in a specific manner.

There were 36 subjects that went through fasting therapy for a time of 10 days and they were re-fed progressively for 5 days afterward. This is compared to the 22 subjects within the control group. The group that did the fasting reported a significant improvement within the symptom levels. These included abdominal pain or discomfort, anorexia, anxiety, and nausea. The other group only included improvements in the levels of bloating and pain. This is a direct connection between intermittent fasting and gut issues and symptoms.

Water fasting has also been said to accelerate healing processes for the gut. Water fasting is where somebody does not consume any food and drinks a lot of water for a period of time. In doing so, they are able to reduce the stress and levels of inflammation within the gut and allowing it to heal and rebuild itself. Fasting also assists to bring down the dysbiotic or microbial growths which are the ones that cause a number of digestive issues. One window of time that seems to provide the majority of the benefits would be between 3 and 5 days. You may start with a 1 day fast. In the event that you do well, then you can go to 2 to 3 days and finally the 3 to 5. A lot of the time, people find when they reach the 3-day period that they get a burst of energy and a lot of mental clarity. This is probably because of entering the ketosis stage where the fats are now burning instead of the glucose. If you feel good on the third day, then it is possible to go up to the fifth day. The maximum for this exercise at a time would probably be up to seven days.

Chapter 9: Intermittent Fasting and Heart Health

Four of the main risks that are related to heart disease would include the likes of cholesterol, diabetes, weight, and blood pressure. The book has already tackled diabetes and cholesterol as well as weight and the contributions that intermittent fasting does to all these risk factors, though there is still the matter of blood pressure and other cardiac injuries. Now, while the effect of human blood pressure levels is not an exact science, there are confirmed studies that have shown that blood pressure reduces in animals during the fasted state and then increases after consumption. There are very few clinical studies that have investigated the effects of intermittent fasting on blood pressure control and the relevant course within patients who are hypertensive.

The only relevant one concerned 174 hypertensive patients that were admitted to a hospital, and they were only issued vegetables and fruit for a period of 2 days. After that, the patients were placed on a water only type of diet which entailed strict fasting up to the point that the blood pressure readings for them had stabilized. Once stable, the patients were placed on a vegan diet that was only vegetables, fruit, and juices, along with a moderate level of exercise. In the results, about 89 percent of the patients had their blood pressure reading show a reduction of both the systolic and diastolic pressure. A lot of the weight loss and the lowering of the levels of blood pressure happened while the patients were on a water only type of diet. The decreasing the blood pressure was most significant in the patients that had a very high blood pressure level.

Cardiac Injuries

Experiments have been done on mice with myocardial infarction and it has been found that intermittent fasting protected the heart from cardiac injury as manifested because of reduced infarctions. These beneficial effects are linked with increased serum adiponectin levels, which have been shown to protect the heart from particular injury. When it comes to the rat model of chronic myocardial ischemia, the intermittent fasting was seen to improve the chances of survival for the subjects when it came to chronic heart failure and also improved the cardiac functions. It resulted in stimulation of angiogenesis and reduced the apoptotic cell denaturing in the border zone of the ischemic hearts.

Intermittent Fasting and Age-Related Hypertrophy

Apparently, intermittent fasting improves the markers for agerelated cardiac hypertrophy and heart failure within the mice such as increased BNP within the heart and the plasma. The advantages of the fasting within the aging heart are attained through bringing back overactivated ERK1/2 and PI3Ky type signaling which are linked to pathological cardiac hypertrophy.

Intermittent Fasting and Coronary Heart Disease Factors

Intermittent fasting is able to change the spectral analysis of blood pressure and the heart rate variability in order to reduce the insulin levels within mice, which are some of the risk factors when it comes to coronary heart disease. Intermittent fasting also allows for lowering of the coronary heart issue risks in people. For example, the intermittent fasting improves the indication of the coronary heart disease in the obese men and women such as body weight, waist circumference, low-density lipoprotein cholesterol, and triacylglycerol. At the same time, intermittent fasting and the manner of calorie restriction with a liquid diet has shown the ability to reduce the factors of coronary heart disease compared with an intermittent fasting restriction without liquid diet in the case of women that are obese. Now, intermittent fasting with high levels of protein and low-calorie type diet reduces the body weight and BMI and also improves the arterial compliance in men and women who are obese. The restriction of heart disease risk factors through the means of intermittent fasting would be linked through the adjusting of adipokines. Clearly, intermittent fasting has been shown to be an asset when it comes to the creation of conditions, which allow for the heart to function beneficially.

It has also been illustrated to create the right situation for healing and the right pressure. There are increasing questions though concerning whether it can lead to side effects which are detrimental to those patients experiencing high blood pressure levels. But clearly, it *is* beneficial.

Chapter 10: Intermittent Fasting and Free Radical Damage

As human beings, everyone requires oxygen in order to survive, but you are still subject to the same oxidation process which in turn causes aging. There is definitely no cure for that, but there is a difference between racing to the finish line and aging gracefully and this is determined by oxidative stress a lot of the time. Oxidative stress, much like in rusting in metals, is a degenerative process that happens because of the imbalance between the production of unstable free radical molecules and the production of antioxidants. A free radical molecule just refers to the molecules that have an unpaired electron, i.e. it can become very reactive.

Basically, the free radical type molecules are going to try and steal one from other healthy cells that are, in turn, going to cause them to become unstable and triggering a chain reaction. The body is going to produce free radical molecules in the event that it counters toxins and other damaging elements including pollution, UV radiation, and pesticides, along with particular ingredients found within the food such as preservatives.

The antioxidants as the name would suggest are those elements which work for the purpose of combating the free radical problems that are in the body. These are compounds which can be created naturally by the body, though the problem is that they are not created in large enough amounts in order to truly combat the issue of oxidative stress. That is the reason why the body is also reliant on a persons diet as antioxidants are usually found within the plant-based foods.

Intermittent fasting could have benefits against oxidative stress. Scientists have been considering the potential health benefits of calorie restriction for some time now. The prominent theory is these health advantages are linked to a drop in the blood sugar which comes from fasting and this pushes the cells in order for them to work that much harder so they can utilize other energy forms. A study done on monkeys, for example, found that if they ate only 70 percent of their normal caloric intake, then they were found to live much longer, and they tended to be healthier during the elderly age groups. These anti-aging benefits have been illustrated as well in animals that went on an intermittent fast as they went between days of normal eating and days when the calories were restricted.

The thing that is not clear though is why intermittent fasting appears to have a benefit when it comes to aging. The question is complicated because, in every research study that was done on people, fasting actually led to weight loss. The benefits of weight loss could be overshadowing the other benefits as attained from solely fasting though.

What is clear is that oxidative stress occurs when there happens to be a higher than normal production of the free radicals like reactive oxygen species. These are some of the unstable molecules which can carry reactive electrons. These would result in a large chain reaction that will go from one molecule to the other and then form free radicals, and these may break the connections between the atoms of significant components within the cellular structure such as the essential proteins, DNA, or the cell membrane. Antioxidants work through the transference of the required electrons in order to stabilize the free radicals before they are able to do any such harm. Even though fasting appears to assist the cells so they can combat the damages occurring from the process, it is yet to be clear on how this occurs.

The free radicals can be generated through mitochondria which are not working in the most effective way. The switch between eating in the normal manner and fasting would cause the cell to temporarily have lower than common levels of blood sugar and they would be forced to start using other sources of energy which are available easily such as fatty acids. This would then cause the cells to begin the survival process which then removes the mitochondria which are not functioning as they should in order to replace them with the healthier options over the course of time. This would result in the reduction of the creation of free radicals over a long time. The other thing is the act of fasting may result in free radical production during the early phases of the exercise. The cells may respond through the increase of the natural antioxidants within the body in order to fight the free radicals. Even though the free radicals are seen as the aggressor considering their ability when it comes to denaturing cells, they could be significant within the short time as they signal the body to trigger cells, so they are better able to adapt in severe stress which may come in the future. This is the case when the body prepares for lean times and adverse weather or environment as if bracing for continuous pain.

Chapter 11: Intermittent Fasting and Epilepsy

Researchers have come to the conclusion that certain diets or patterns of eating are effective when it comes to the treatment of epilepsy through finding that the metabolism of particular neural cells affects the way they can send information. The connections between these cellular processes, which were at one time assumed not to be related, open the avenue for the treatment of epilepsy without a need for medication that is not pleasant.

Even before the anti-convulsion medications were created during the 1950s, the epileptics would try and reduce their diet as a means of limiting the seizures that they had. In fact, the ancients in Greece came to realize that the periods related to fasting would make the seizures become less frequent and they would also lose their severity. The bible is also fond of using fasting for various treatments of conditions to do with spirituality so it would make sense that fasting also helped with several physical issues. During the early 1900s, a number of epileptic patients even resorted to the keto diet because it was thought to imitate the physiological effects which would arrive with fasting. There are several experts who have confirmed that the diet restrictions may trigger some chemical changes which short-circuit some of the parts of the brain thus initiating the levels of the seizures. Though, the mechanism which is behind the therapeutic effects would still be a bit mysterious.

Within the current study, the researchers have considered the neurons which do not allow for activity since the drugs which treat epilepsy function through the strengthening of the ability of the brain when it comes to shutting things down whenever it is about to lose control. Dr. Derek Bowie from McGill University took the time to explain that the pharmacological approaches may have some disadvantages considering the patients likely complain about unpleasant side effects. Apparently, about 20 to 30 percent of patients that have epilepsy do not respond well to drug medication and this could provide an explanation as to why the keto diet became quite popular up until intermittent fasting.

Overall, the study was illustrative that the brain has an inbuilt remedy which was to deal with overactivity that could be harnessed with the appropriate dietary consideration. Since the study shows brain cells have a way to strengthen inhibition, the work then illustrates new means of controlling a number of neurological conditions such as epilepsy. There has been a long assumption that intermittent fasting reduces the levels of seizures through affecting a similar type of mechanism. Research is increasingly proving that the two approaches operate differently and so they can be used in tandem in order to have a better control of the seizures. This is particularly relevant when it comes to the children suffering from epilepsy.

Chapter 12: Intermittent Fasting, Cancer, and Diabetes

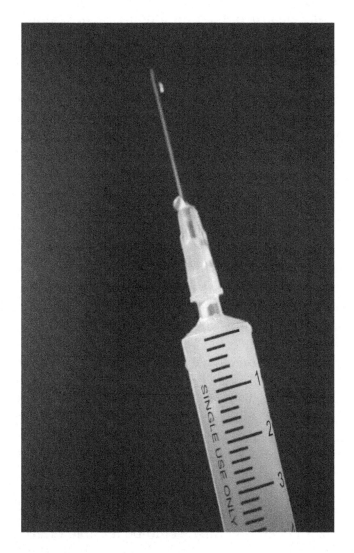

The main health benefit that has been discussed with intermittent fasting is weight loss, longevity, and epilepsy, however, there are other considerations worth mentioning such as cancer and diabetes. Research is increasingly proving that

there are several benefits to this diet that go beyond weight loss.
This includes the lowering levels of blood sugar and the assistance in the reduction of the resistance to insulin and leptin. Fasting has also been illustrated to improve cardiovascular health and to promote neural development.

Triggering of the Immune System in Patients

One of the ways which the fasting diet would assist people suffering from cancer would be through triggering the immune system. The immune system is designed in a way that it looks for and kills pathogens that are considered harmful to the body. However, it appears to be less able in doing its job with the abnormal cells within the body. Many cancer treatments are being developed for the purpose of stimulating the immune system so that it can do this but the present research is coming up with a fasting mode which would assist in doing the same task. One particular study from the University of Southern California was done with the use of lab mice and it came to the conclusion that when mice received chemotherapy and a fasted diet, the immune system was then able to look for and kill the breast and skin cancer cells. The lab mice were able to produce more immune system cells when they were on a fast including T cells and B cells which were better at actively targeting and eliminating the tumor cells. The other realization was the cells which usually protect the tumors known as the T regulatory cells were kept outside of the tumors. And that they may have assisted the chemotherapy drugs, so they could work better.

The same authors of the study advanced the research to a pilot survey with human cancer patients in order to see if the diets combined with chemotherapy would be feasible or even safe to conduct and whether it would be beneficial for the recovery process. In this case, the water-only two-day fast and a four-day fast with restricted calorie diet which imitates fasting was found to be safe for the cancer patients under the doctor's supervision. All of the conclusions on these matters were an indication that a fasting diet and chemotherapy could be utilized in order to slow the rate of tumor growth in cancer patients.

Efficacy in Animal Testing

In several findings for animal studies, the fasting appeared both to reduce the levels of toxicity and increase the efficacy of chemotherapy. It seems that when the normal cells are deprived of nutrients, they would be protected from chemotherapy while dividing the cancer cells in order for them to expend energy while starving and so they are more susceptible to attack through the means of chemotherapy. At the same time, fasting reduces protein kinase A (PKA) activation and increases the activated protein kinase activity. These signal transductions which lead to particular changes and then cause the activation of the early growth-response type proteins.

Even though animal testing is proving to be promising, the question is whether the results can be translated for human beings as well. In a situation report consisting of 10 patients being treated for different cancers, the ones that did a water-fast with vitamins for a period of between 48 and 140 hours before and 5 to 56 hours after chemotherapy reported there was a bigger tolerance for treatment. They also did not have any weakness or gastrointestinal symptoms as compared to the previous nonfasting type treatments.

Fasting also did not seem to prevent the chemotherapy-induced shrinkage of the tumors or affect the markers. There were admittedly some minor complaints such as dizziness and headaches but it was at such a level that it would not interfere with daily activities. Two years ago, a study that entailed 20 patients receiving platinum-based regimens entailed them fasting for three days, which was 48 hours of prechemotherapy and 24 hours of post-chemotherapy. The patients were made to consume as little calories as possible and they had to drink water. In the event symptoms related to fasting occurred such as weakness, then they would be allowed to consume a small amount of juice or even food. There were no grade 3 toxicities that were realized though because of the fast and the lab studies that were done on the matter did not reveal any evidence of malnutrition. The researchers cautioned though on the safety of fasting before chemotherapy. The patients that would not be ideal would be those who had already experienced more than 10 percent loss in their body weight or had a BMI of less than 20.5.

Randomized trials in animals have been there in order to determine the effect of fasting on cancer treatment efficiency and other problematic effects. Now, the experiments are slowly but gradually moving to human subjects. Experts at certain clinics are already enrolling patients for clinical trials in order to evaluate the safety and feasibility of short-term periods of fasting prior to the administration of chemotherapy. They are also evaluating the effects of fasting on the weight change in order to determine the longest possible fasting period before chemotherapy. Though, from the evidence available in most animal trials along with the ones which have been done on people, it would seem there is a beneficial effect to fasting during cancer treatment which has created unproven claims like fasting will treat cancer or even prevent a recurrence of the condition.

Calorie Restriction, Fasting, and Cancer

In 2013, the oncologist magazine commented in the editorial concerning research from Chicago which illustrated that restriction of the calorie intake in patients doing radiotherapy resulted in better results. In 2018, there was some evidence revealed which illustrated chemotherapy increased the levels of inflammation within the body and that reducing intake of calories had the ability in order to effectively reduce this.

This is contrary to the booklets claiming that you can pour dairy and starch into your system when undergoing chemotherapy. In fact, you are more than likely adding fuel to cancer that is eating you alive. More reviews and research studies come out every month on the subject even though it may not be particular conditions, but the consensus is that fasting may improve the efficiency of chemotherapy in putting cancer into remission. It may even allegedly reduce the side effects. The theory is simple. Fasting causes a signal to be issued to the cells through the sirtuin hormones in order to make them shut down. Their metabolic rate would then decline in order for them not to take on board the chemotherapy, which leaves more of the cancer cells that are metabolizing in a vigorous manner.

The theory has been tested by Longo in mice in 2008 and was proven correct on a number of additions. Fasting alone apparently caused the cancer building blocks and infected cells to self-destruct. That is, they did not understand the message to shut down and so they had to keep metabolizing but there were no nutrients and this resulted in the death of the cancer cells within the research. The other thing was the tumor activity not only went down but the aggression of the tumors also reduced on a significant level. In the tests which included mice, a fifth of the ones with metastasis which fasted and underwent chemotherapy were cured while 40 percent stopped their cancerous progression. It is now widely accepted among various advocates of fasting that it is better to fast for a period of 2 to 3 days before the chemo.

How to Fast During Cancer Treatments

It does not matter whether you are a disciple of the Longo approach or are undergoing chemotherapy; you ought to go on a water fast for 3 to 5 days as the maximum. This type of fast would bring plasma glucose and even the insulin levels to nil. It would also bring down the amino acids levels and stop the progression of cancer while stopping metastases and making the chemo that much more effective while helping to restart the immune system. Though, if the water fast is too extreme, then various intermittent fast models would suffice such as the warrior diet or up day down day fasts. These fasts that used over two to three weeks at a time *do* reduce the levels of cholesterol and triglycerides and they even reduce diabetes, which will be covered in the next section of the chapter. If you do not have diabetes, then a non-starchy organic vegetable juice diet for a time of 3 to 5 days would also present a viable option for the patient.

Considering Treatment Options

Various cancer specialists have considered the dangers to do with weight loss on account of cachexia with regards to the intermittent fast routine. Cachexia is a deterioration of tissues disorder which is an indication of cancer, AIDS, or even heart disappointment that accompanies side effects including muscle loss, the absence of craving, weakness, and diminished quality dimensions. Despite the fact that this is an alternate issue as it relates uncontrolled weight loss caused by reactions of chemotherapy and symptoms like nausea bringing about the decrease of cravings. This is not really a controlled weight loss but a medication incited kind of disease. Research done on patients doing chemotherapy has demonstrated that omega 3 from fish may help patients to recover their hunger and their weight. The equivalent might be valid for various cancers, however, eating awful fats has been connected to bring down rates of survival in ladies experiencing cervical and bosom cancers yet eating characteristic or immersed fats has been connected to expanded rates of recuperation and survival. This is a full invert of the NHS exhortation to patients to expend as many calories as could reasonably be expected while experiencing chemotherapy.

Evidently, the national cancer institute is exceptionally intrigued by fasting as they think about that the food that a person eats may influence the way that the body assimilates and responds to the treatment choices or the medications. For them, fasting could be some method for helping chemotherapy to think of better outcomes with fewer reactions and more expense adequately. Dr. Longo, for instance, exhibited that fasting for a period of a few days ensured the solid cells in societies with cancer tumors from chemotherapy drugs without securing the cancer cells themselves. Researchers also conducted an investigation of 10 elderly patients who willfully experienced fasting for a brief span when they attempted chemotherapy. The patients at that point detailed a lower dimension of reactions. Because of contentions that fasting would advance the dimensions of cancer growth, a similar group thought of research representing fasting makes the cancer cells more vulnerable to chemotherapy. Fasting really prevented the cancer cells from creating assurance proteins from the transformed qualities while eating well cells brought about proteins that are more protective. The outcome was that sound cells quit isolating yet they likewise get less assaulted by the chemo thus there are lesser antagonistic symptoms. In a few mixes of chemo and fasting, the tumors vanished even. The group identified a second factor that was neutralizing the cancer cells. Fasting deprived the cancer of glucose. These have been considered as stressors representing the upgrading of cancer.

Intermittent Fasting and Diabetes

It has already been established that intermittent fasting is good for the heart, weight loss, and the reduction of blood pressure over some periods. These would all probably be seen to contribute to creating an environment where it would be hard to develop diabetes within the system since it already reduces the levels of blood sugar.

There is also a lot of research presently which shows that intermittent fasting when it comes to type 2 diabetes, would assist with the reduction of insulin resistance which is a big problem with people that are suffering from the condition.

While not addressed in the diabetes guidelines, intermittent fasting is a meal timing type of approach which could help prediabetic individuals achieve and maintain weight loss levels and a better control of insulin sensitivity. One of the attractive elements when it comes to intermittent fasting for assisting in the prevention of diabetes is that it considers a relatively simple intervention for people and their families to take on. The practice of intermittent fasting is made even better at this day and age considering the mobile apps available to help the person keep track and share their meal timing with friends and family in order to gain social support in the process.

In this way, those who are at risk or with pre-diabetes are then able to restrict their calories naturally and even to a point that it is no longer intentional. According to a study that was done in 2014 with 54 volunteers (that had type 2 diabetes), the participants that only ate breakfast and lunch had better increases in their insulin sensitivity and they reduced body weight, not to mention the levels of blood sugar. This is compared to the patients that ate smaller meals during the day as people are able to cut their intake of calories without the psychological and physiological stress of keeping a food journal.

On the other hand, there have not been a lot of rigorous studies concerning intermittent fasting in the participants that have type 2 diabetes and low blood sugar symptoms. Additional research pieces are therefor needed for the purpose of learning the benefits of fasting not to mention the potential problems that would arrive with them. Intermittent fasting without the right supervision could be a problem for some people with diabetes particularly the ones that use hypoglycemic medications in the process.

A randomized trial that was published in a renowned journal, Diabetic Medicine came to the realization that 5:2 intermittent fasting which includes two consecutive or non-consecutive days of fasting followed by five days of regular calorie intake every week is then linked to mild increases in hypoglycemia in the case of diabetes on hypoglycemic medication. On the other hand, the study also found that as long as patients get guidance and education on the reduction of medication for fasting days, alternate day fasting could be relatively safe and effective when it comes to weight loss, improved blood sugar control, and improved fasting glucose levels.

The individuals with diabetes need to consult with their primary care physicians before they embark on trying any intermittent fasting schedule to come up with an individualized meal timing and medication reduction plan. Soon, particular apps are going to assist patients in doing this by allowing the patients to share data with and get notifications from their health care providers. The timing of the insulin resistance measurements may affect the results.

After the end of a 36-hour fast, a person would appear to be more insulin-resistant than if they were measured after 24 hours of fasting. In order to assess the insulin resistance, there is a need to consider the whole 24-hour profile. According to some researchers, there seem to be a number of reasons why animals such as rats, in particular, would suffer from the problem of intermittent fasting. For one, it could be because of protein deficiencies. A number of studies of intermittent fasting in rodents have come up with positive results so the readers need to take the major points concerning the particular study with a grain of salt so to speak.

Timing Is Everything

Another pilot study concerning intermittent fasting in individuals with type 2 diabetes revealed intermittent fasting would be a safe and simple dietary intervention for improving the body weight, fasting glucose, and blood sugar control. The participants of the study apparently fasted for a time of 18 hours each day and they basically started eating in the early afternoon thereafter. By having the participants take photos of their meals previously and after eating, the researchers came to know that intermittent fasting leads to a spontaneous yet an overall decrease within the calorie intake. The participants that fasted for 18 hours each day felt things like weight loss as well as improved morning fasted levels of blood sugar along with postmeal high blood sugar levels.

The pilot study concerning time-restricted feeding in diabetics did not find any incidences of hypoglycemia. Even though the intervention only lasted for a period of two weeks and the individuals self-reported their blood sugar levels and eating hours, the researchers observed many improvements in diabetic glucose control. Several small-scale key studies have showed that the animals and humans, when it came to intermittent fasting regimens ranging from the time restricted feeding to alternate day fasting, experience a number of improvements when it comes to metabolic health. Longo, for example, published a study where 100 healthy individuals ate a calorie-restricted diet for a time of 5 days every month. The subjects began with high blood sugar experienced significant advancements and none of the subjects experienced harmful effects. Fasting, for one, reduced the body weight level and lowered the blood pressure, as did fasting glucose, triglycerides and higher risks for diabetes. Thus, there is a need for more human clinical trial research to learn the impacts and safety for a number of the fasting regiments concerning the diabetes risk indicators. Not every one of the intermittent fasting regimens is equal and moderate when it comes to time restricted schedules after all. However, there is a lot of evidence suggesting that daytime time-regulated consumption could be the simplest and effective step for prediabetes and type-2 diabetes. Patients should try these out for health purposes so long as they work with a physician in order to monitor the levels of blood sugar and to monitor their medications in the right manner.

Possible Downsides

The biggest downside when it comes to intermittent fasting for the people that have type 2 diabetes is the ganger that comes with low blood sugar. For these particular seasons, it would be recommended that the diabetics that wish to follow the diets consult with a nutritionist of their healthcare practitioner in order to carefully monitor the levels of sugars to adjust medications in the event that the low blood sugar is an issue. In a recent study, the participants who numbered 37 were divided into two groups. One of them fasted for two days that were not consecutive, and the other fasted on two consecutive days over a period of 12 weeks. There were various progressions seen in the level of weight, fasting glucose, and the quality of life for each participant with an average rate of 1.4 hypoglycemic events for the ones on medications that produced hypoglycemia. The occasional skipped meal supposedly would not cause an issue for the majority of people with type 2 diabetes apparently. According to Mario Skugor, a clinical assistant and professor of medicine at an endocrine and metabolic clinic in Cleveland, there shouldn't be a reason that weight loss would be an issue, though if the patient was on a sulfonylurea, then skipping meals would allegedly cause a state of low blood sugar.

On the other hand, there was another study which found advantages for people living with type 2 diabetes. Three men between the ages of 40 and 67 tried doing intermittent fasting so they could see if it would improve the state of their health and reduce the reliance they had on medication and insulin. The men, in this case, had suffered from diabetes for varying amounts of time from the time they were 10 to even from the time some were young adults. They had also been taking various drugs in order to control their disease and daily insulin amounts. In addition to diabetes, they were all suffering from high cholesterol levels and high blood pressure levels as well. One of the men had fasted for three days each week while the other two had fasted on alternate days for a period of 24 hours. During the fast days, they were allowed to take in liquids such as water, broth, and one low-calorie level meal during the dinner time. They had all participated in a 6-hour nutritional training seminar as well so they could educate themselves on the way diabetes developed and its effect on their systems not to mention how they could manage their conditions through the means of diet.

In less than one year after embarking on their fasting routine, the average levels of AIC, weight and waist circumference had dropped significantly to manageable levels. Each of the three was also able to stop doing insulin injections within a month after beginning on their fasting schedules. In one of the cases, he only had to do so after a time of five days. Two of the men were also able to stop taking medication and the third man discounted at least three of the four medications that he had been taking the whole time.

Intermittent Fasting and Its Effect on Blood Sugar Control

The main worry of most experts when it comes to intermittent fasting probably has to do with the blood sugar control. For one, skipping entire meals when it comes to intermittent fasting can result in a more negative effect on the level of blood glucose control as well as problems such as fatigue and low levels of energy when you are exercising not to mention imbalances brought by medication within the system. On a psychological front, it can also lead to worse diet choices having the opposite effect on the waistline and blood sugar levels. Those people that restrict their calories could be more inclined to reach for heavy carb diets on their off days depending on the type of intermittent fast they may go for. This would be a yo-yo effect from having to starve themselves during the fast. The thing that most do not realize is just because there is an opportunity provided by the fast to eat during a 6-hour period, it does not mean gulping down anything and everything that they can get their hands on.

As such, severe restriction of the calories or even skipping them altogether can be hard as a schedule for someone to stick to. It would seem the problem with fasting is it is much harder for a person to adopt as a lifestyle in the long term. Though losing weight can be a great benefit for people that are suffering from diabetes as it increases the insulin sensitivity, putting weight back on may have the opposite effect and as a result increase the risk of diabetes complications. At the same time, there are certain factors such as breastfeeding moms or those who are pregnant. In fact, at any time that one wants or needs a high level of nutrition, it would not be advisable for them to begin intermittent fasting.

In the case of pregnant women, they need the extra calories for them and their children. Fasting can lead them to dangerous levels of blood sugar. The other thing is if a pregnant mother overproduces ketones, the effect may be harmful to the baby. Similarly, for someone that has an overactive thyroid, intermittent fasting may lead to something which is known as a thyroid storm which causes increases in temperature not to mention a rapid heart rate and even heart problems. The other problem for people suffering from diabetes would be low blood sugar. In a study done in 2016, there were 150 participants that fasted on a regular basis and 10 percent of these individuals experienced hypoglycemia. The people that are on particular diabetic medications or insulin especially could be at risk of the complications which could end up being life-threatening.

Considering the dangers brought by blood sugar fluctuation that could be initiated by intermittent fasting, some experts advocate against this diet plan for those who have type 2 diabetes. The highs and lows appear to be the main risk as they may lead to complications and critical conditions of the patients. The apparent objective when it comes to diabetes would be maintaining a steady blood sugar level during the whole day allegedly. Apparently, diabetics also have the risk of contracting diabetic ketoacidosis that is a complication which happens when the body is not able to produce enough insulin.

Insulin is what brings glucose within the cells when the body does not have enough of it because the carbohydrates are not available during the fasting time, and then the body ends up overproducing ketones. These ketones are there because of the fats burned to produce energy but they build up in the system. The result is they may damage the kidneys and go to the brain causing brain swelling.

Diabetic ketoacidosis is quite serious if not taken care of and could even lead to diabetic coma or may be fatal. For anyone, in spite of whether they have diabetes, cutting out the meals and restricting food groups can increase the chances of causing nutritional deficiencies. Without the right amount of nutrients, especially protein, then there may be a risk of muscle mass loss.

Hence, the thing is to keep your expectations in check when it comes to diabetes though this would also apply to others who approach intermittent fasting as a fix all remedy. Intermittent fasting as a plan does not work for everyone and the medical team that you consult with may not feel that it is a good idea in your case. It would be important to consult your assigned professionals before going into intermittent fasting especially if you have type-2 diabetes because going for long periods without consuming anything while with the condition may be a bit dangerous or at the least will not produce the results that you want. If you are recommending something to the patient, then you will have to consider the whole picture and consider if it would fit within your life and if the results are of more significance than the risks.

Together with your doctor, you can decide on what is sustainable and within your best interests. Because of the risk that comes with potential blood sugar swings, full-blown intermittent fasting may not be the appropriate option for someone that is suffering from diabetes. One option if you still want to wing it though may be decreasing the portion of food that you eat at a go and increase the frequency of physical activity between meals. You may also opt to make healthy food swaps that align with intermittent fasting which will make it a better approach.

Chapter 13: Understanding Food Proteins, Carbs, and Fats

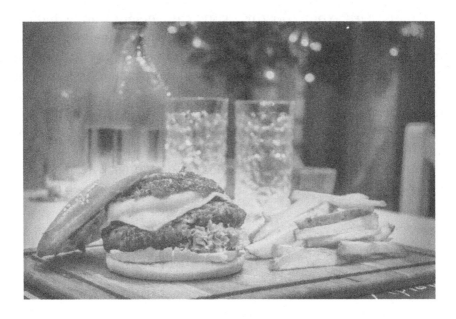

Intermittent fasting should be looked at as a strategy rather than a diet because it is a strategy that aims at your fat stores. If your overall goal is to lose weight, then you can proceed with a calorierestrictive diet. Intermittent fasting allows the practitioner some control over their meals and cravings. So, when you fast for a time of between 8 to 12 hours, the levels of insulin in the bloodstream drop and the body will start to tap into the fat stores rather than the carbs. This then asks the question of how much carbs can you eat during the time of fasting.

A number of sources claim that you should aim to make 35 to 40 percent of the calories taken during the eating period carbs, and the rest would be protein and fat. From a diet of 2,000 to 2,500 calories, that would mean a maximum of 1,000 calories in a day. So, in a sense, that would tell you that there is no big restriction or diet to intermittent fasting but instead is a particular *schedule*. The other approach you can take with carbs during intermittent fasting is carb cycling. Long-term restriction of carbs may lower the metabolic rates and negatively affect the levels of your hormones, though it can also be of benefit. Carb cycling allows for planned high carb days that increase the thyroid output and allows you to control your hunger. Because you will be cycling your carbs, there will also be low-carb days that offset the high carb days.

With that cycle, it will be possible for you to continue seeing fat loss, increased levels of energy, and improvements to your overall body structure. Carb cycling improves the levels of insulin and assists the body to burn more fat.

Intermittent Fasting Meets Carb Cycling

Carb cycling is not for everyone and I personally don't use this method as I find it to be too restrictive on my lifestyle. I don't like to place a lot of rules on the way I eat as I will tell you about later in the different types of fasting section. I will explain what it's all about anyway for those interested there are certain parameters when it comes to intermittent fasting carb cycling as a plan each week, for example, you can choose three low-carb days, one high carb day and three moderate levels of carb days. The days you set these up on are not relevant and it is also possible for you to change those days on the go. For example, you might have a date or some other type of event that might influence you to make that particular day the high carb one. The days when you are working and do not have time for food could then become be the low-carb days.

During the low-carb days, you may have around 0.25 - 0.5 grams of carbs per pound of body weight, this is a general number as it can also depend if you are applying a certain diet such as the Keto or paleo diets to your intermittent fasting lifestyle.

During the moderate carb days, you could consume around 0.5 - 1 gram of carbs per pound of body weight. During the weekly high carb days, it is possible to eat as many carbs as possible, obviously making sure you get your stick to your protein and fat amounts would keep this number from getting out of control.

With your carbs set for each day of the week, the other considerations to fit into the diet equation would be the protein and fat. Anyone that knows anything about building muscle knows that proteins are the building blocks for muscle fiber. It goes without saying that you need to get an adequate amount of protein into you during your feeding window. Every day, regardless if you are carb cycling and are on your low, moderate or high carb day it would is super important that you get enough protein. I recommend around 0.82 – 1 gram of protein for per pound of body weight, so that means if you weigh 150 pounds that's around 123 - 150 grams of protein per day. Protein is particularly important for intermittent fasting concerning the first meal after the fast.

One of the main ways to make intermittent fasting work, after all, is to boost the metabolism. Low metabolism makes the cells less efficient when it comes to deriving of energy so that more protein and fat would be burned for a similar amount of energy. Fat is also crucial for building muscle and maintaining while aiding the levels of fat loss. You can aim for around 0.5 grams of healthy fats per pound of body weight every day. That would imply eating half of your body weight in grams in terms of fat.

If intermittent fasting allows the individual to fit the diet into their lifestyle and stick to it, then that is commendable. The great thing about the intermittent carb cycle is it is easy for you to prevent yourself from going overboard and shooting over your macros.

It takes a bit of thought and some planning to do, though. For example, on a Friday or Saturday, you may have a date and you know there is going to be a temptation to eat something fatty and heavy on the carbs. The best thing to do in this situation is to cut the feeding window back so the only food for the day would be that meal or outing. That way, even if you exceed one or two macros, you will be under on another one. The other thing is the extra time spent fasting is going to further prevent damage from some extra fat and carbs for the night. You may also change the feeding and fasting windows according to what you may need to train or eat on a particular day. For example, you may start the feeding window at 4 PM because you train after this period but at one time, you may need to do so three hours earlier. You may start eating at 1 PM which is three hours earlier than the standard. You should not crucify yourself for not having lasted the full 16 hours for the fast so give some leeway for the diet but do not make it a habit.

Looking out for the Plateau

One of the great things when it comes to carb cycling is it assists you in preventing the plateau area where fat loss stops completely. The thing with dieting and weight loss is your body hates change, it loves to stay in that comfort zone and resists being inconvenienced and going into nutrient deficiency. That means when the calories go down for a certain amount of time, your metabolism also drops so that you can run on a smaller amount of calories. When this is the case, the fat loss slows down or it even stops all together. When you finally hit a plateau, the only means to continue with the loss of fat is dropping the calories, now obviously you can only continue to drop your calories for so long before it becomes dangerous. However, through cycling your carbs and calories, your body still does not adapt as fast to the new amounts of calories and this is good when it comes to losing as much fat as possible. You might find that you can keep to the diet plan as outlined for some time before hitting the plateau. Now, if the plateau has arrived, the best strategy would just be to reduce the number of days where you consume the moderate amounts of carbs. You might notice fat loss stalls after a number of months following carb cycling under intermittent fasting. In order to proceed with fat loss after this occurs, it is advisable to turn one moderate carb day each week so that it becomes a low-carb day for a small period like a month to shock your body and give it something it's not use to before going back to what you were doing.

Chapter 14: Satiety and Binge Eating

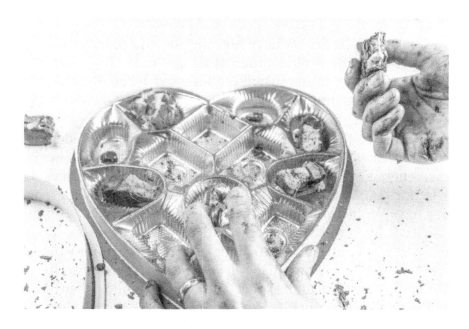

Intermittent fasting challenges our discipline and allows us to seek methods of controlling ourselves so that we stick to a particular feeding pattern for the sake of health, mentally and emotionally speaking. As such, the people who take on this approach have to rewire how they perceive hunger and cravings, and in a way, they have to restructure their relationship with food. The poor relationships that people have with food come to the surface in the form of binge and emotional eating.

Binge eating refers to a person who has lost control of themselves and then takes in a large amount of food and as a result ends up overeating without a second thought or being able to stop. This is very closely related to obesity and certain behaviors. Emotional eating, on the other hand, is the consumption of food as a response to emotional trauma. If a person has ever overeaten in order to suppress feelings of guilt or sadness, then they know what emotional eating is like. Emotional eating similarly is linked with poor diet, greater intake of energy dense foods, along with sweet and high-fat snacks not to mention lower fruit and vegetable intake.

Traditionally, physicians have not had the equipment to assist their people with problematic eating patterns. Bingeing and emotional eating is not usually addressed when it comes to weight loss programs as well.

In response to the modern cultural trends leading to sedentary lifestyles involving processed foods and fast foods, health researchers have considered simple intervention techniques. In order for people to attain much better relationships with food, they need intermittent fasting. These interventions can be practiced by almost everyone with the exception of those suffering from particular nutritional issues or pregnant women. But even people who are diabetic or cancerous can subscribe to this eating pattern and expect successful results when their medication is also considered as a factor.

Intuitive eating is a term that was initiated in 1995 and encourages a heightened level of awareness when it comes to physical hunger and a simple yet consistent approach for eating healthily. Eating in an intuitive manner apparently means staying away from yo-yo dieting patterns. It allows for the ideology that no particular food type is bad for you but needs to be approached with an element of moderation. As such, it has been linked with a decreased risk of cardiovascular disease and BMI, not to mention a higher level of awareness for physical hunger cues and pleasure which is associated with the food.

The addition of meditation to the intuitive eating approach has gained a lot of traction recently thus resulting in a number of mindful eating training programs and research studies on the subject. The interventions for mindful eating have also shown there are positive effects on binge eating and emotional eating. There have also been illustrated positive effects on obesity and behaviors related to it. Mindful eating as a technique for intermittent fasting and this leads to the initiative of the means to break bad relationships with food.

Breaking Bad Eating Habits Utilizing Intermittent Fasting

When you are discussing eating habits particularly within the fitness population, the subject is very sensitive. For a lot of people, eating is more than a task that is done for survival. It is an enjoyable thing that most people look forward to and no matter what people might say it is addictive. Only for very few people, is it treated as a way to supply the body its need for energy. For the rest, the best way to go about restructuring your thoughts on eating includes rethinking hunger and certain reactions.

False Hunger Cues

People are generally creatures of habit, so they get used to a particular schedule when it comes to certain dietary habits. These habits are looked at as acceptable or not depending on your perception as well as your objectives or beliefs on the subject. Unfortunately, for most people in the modern cultures of the west and even the east, the common diet is lacking when it is compared to a diet of fresh and unprocessed food. As a result, those people who are unhappy and overweight usually have eating habits which they have lost control of. This concerns their selection of what to eat and the frequency of their eating habits.

Their rate of intake tends to be high-calorie type foods and they eat as often as possible due to false hunger cues. If somebody gets used to eating eight meals in a day then suddenly goes to three, their body will issue signals of hunger even though it has all the nutrients it needs from the three meals given that day. This is the result of being dependent on certain processed foods that are addictive yet offer little or no nutritional value other than being carb filled for energy but even then, they come with numerous additives which counteract this benefit.

Relearn the True Meaning of Hunger

The question becomes how you actually relearn what hunger is like. The best answer is not to eat for some time. If you would like to relearn what true hunger feels like, the appropriate thing to do is go on a 24-hour fast. By the time that it is over, you will be hungry but it will not be based on a craving for food but for nutrients. You may feel starved for sustenance though in the real sense of the word you are not there yet. You just are not used to not having something to eat.

Hunger pangs within the body are mostly controlled through hormones such as leptin and ghrelin. This means that when a person is used to eating several times during the day and are on a constant sugar rush, the hunger pangs are going to be at a high. This is supposedly a good thing. In order to change a person's bad eating habits, they have to re-train themselves to learn what true hunger feels like. Once this happens, then you will need to be reminded of what being full feels like.

Making Yourself Full

The state of being full possesses different meanings for different people. For some people that eat slowly, it is the second that their neural system or brain receives the signal that they are full. At this time, they stop eating even if their plate has food on it. For other people that eat quite fast, this would be after they consume the fourth plate of food in front of them even if their bodies signaled they were full at the third one. The thing is they ate so fast that the feeling of hunger did not fully show up until the time they were on the fourth plate. As a result, by this time, they would need somewhere to rest so that the body processes all the food.

For the people that eat more than they should, there is a need to find a medium. This should also be dependent on the amount of physical exercise that they perform each day. If the energy requirements are for somebody to sit at their desk for more than ten hours, then the portions of food should be small and reduced in the carb department. It is a different case if the person is in a field which entails a lot of movement such as the military or if they are a mechanic or work with their hands. At the same time, they can also attempt drinking lots of water in between meals. You should also avoid or change the focus in the way that you perceive marketing for processed food as a direct link to health problems.

If you see the McDonald's package in that way, it is going to be hard for you to binge eat after a long day. You may also try high saturated fat diets at the end of a fast which make you feel satiated and are less prone to make you dependent.

Principles to Feeling Satiated

When relearning a good way to feeling full, you can go about it a few ways. You can stick with whole foods only and eat only 1 or two meals every day depending on the structure of the intermittent fast. On the days which you are more active, you may have bigger portions during the meals and lesser portions when you are sedentary. There are a couple of things to think about when satiety is the main priority.

- Eating protein in each meal: It is the most satisfying component and would lead to better muscle mass. When organizing the meal, I would suggest that it is set at a higher portion level, like 35 percent of the meal.

- Eating fiber-rich vegetables: These are especially low in calories and they give a considerable quantity to the eating regimen considering their content of minerals and fiber.
- Fruit rather than carbs: The water and the fiber content inside these foods will leave you feeling full for a longer time when contrasted with bread or oats.

- Eating more fat: Fat is satisfying; however, it is very easy for someone to overindulge on the portions for it. Some examples of for this would be nut butter or cooking semi cuts of red meats.

Feasting After the Fast

Self-control is very significant when it comes to making sure that a person follows the rules of the fast. The greatest struggle when it comes to intermittent fasting is not just the fast itself but the way it is broken. This is so that you do not end up overindulging and turning around the benefits your body has received up until that point. You will feel hunger and will lead to cravings since you are not used to going this long without eating something. A great deal of self-discipline will prove to be useful at some point.

You also have to eat appropriate quantities, which will lead to satiety instead of stuffing yourself just to feel hopeless after breaking the fast. There is no reason for you to go on a full-scale binge and pig out as much as possible just because you were in a fast. This is counterproductive to your goals. In fact, if you have the tendency to binge-eat right after fasts, then you may need to deal with that problem before starting off on the fast because little or no progress will be made with that process.

You will likewise need to monitor the calories in a similar manner as you would with different weight control plans like the Atkins or the Keto Diet. In this case, you need to keep it inside the slated 2,000 to 2,500 calories. In any case, the great thing with intermittent fasting is that it makes the eating regimen easy and enables you to understand what it feels like to feel satisfied and listen out for genuine hunger cues instead of the false ones.

However, if you feel intermittent fasting does not fit within your schedule, I would highly recommend you give it a go anyway, I can't stress how effective this method is in achieving the body you have always wanted. It will only take a time of three to four weeks for you to relearn hunger pangs while on the intermittent fast and get back on track. Once a grip has been attained on the schedule, then it will be easy for you to eat out of necessity as opposed to other reasons.

Intermittent fasting is definitely not for the faint of heart. It is a lifestyle change-program meant to re-orient the way you see food. Food should not be addictive but rather more on the functional side. On the plus side, this is one of the ways you can build up your self-discipline.

Chapter 15: IF For Woman

Specific Effects of Intermittent Fasting on the Female Body And Precautions For Potential Hazards.

So far we have gone through exactly what intermittent fasting is, as well as some of the many benefits you can expect to experience while following this dietary lifestyle. While the effects that we discussed are the same for both men and women, this chapter is about intermittent fasting for women. Therefore, we will focus on effects of intermittent fasting more specific to the female body. Furthermore, while there are many benefits that women can reap from choosing to fast, there are also some health concerns unique to women that we should discuss, as well as how you can avoid them. After all, if you choose to begin intermittent fasting to live a healthier and fuller life, the last thing you want is to create new health problems in the process!

We have discussed how intermittent fasting can help both men and women lose weight, have more energy, and even lower their risks for many types of diseases. However, there have been numerous studies performed using only women as subjects where intermittent fasting has proven extremely effective at providing these benefits. A study published in the International Journal of Obesity in 2011 selected two groups of women and subjected them to two different methods of fasting, continuous (no food for an entire day) and intermittent. While both groups of women lost weight, the group that adhered to intermittent fasting saw 30% of the women losing anywhere from 5-10% of their body weight, and 34% of these women lost over 10% of their body weight.

What is even more remarkable about these findings is that these women were not instructed to exercise, and made little if any changes in their amount of physical activity during this study.

We are not talking about a few pounds here and there, without even taking exercise into consideration, these women were able to lose a remarkable amount of body weight by just trying intermittent fasting. While this study was performed to see how fasting affected weight loss in women, researchers also wanted to see if this lifestyle was really effective in preventing certain diseases. They measured certain risk markers for things such as diabetes, cancer, and cardiovascular disease in these women before the study began, and immediately afterwards. What they found was that after following the intermittent fasting protocol, these risk markers were decreased substantially in all of the women.

Another study published in the Nutrition Journal in 2012 aimed to learn what happened to the energy needs in the female body when fasting begins. A group of women were selected to follow an 8-week, calorie restricted intermittent fasting plan. What they found was that the women's bodies actually had a huge reduction in their body's energy needs, between 75-90%. Intermittent fasting makes the female body incredibly more efficient and teaches it to use energy much more effectively. Once again, the human body is an incredible piece of machinery, and is extremely adaptive and knows how to maintain itself at all costs. When it experiences fasting, it will teach itself to run just as well, if not even better on fewer calories, as it plunges into fat reserves to continue functioning optimally.

Now there are a few health concerns specific to the female body that I would like to address when it comes to intermittent fasting. The first of these are drastic hormonal food cravings, there are numerous hormones in the body that regulate and control hunger. These include insulin, leptin, and ghrelin, among many others. Women subjected to extended periods of fasting (as in not eating for an entire day) are susceptible to having these hormones thrown out of whack.

When this happens, the chemical signals in the brain that let you know when you are full and should not eat anymore become turned off, which can cause overeating. A study consisting of female college students at the University of Virginia had the subjects fast for two whole days. What they found was that levels of leptin in these women decreased by as much as 75%! This can severely disrupt feelings of satiety and result in someone consuming entirely too many calories when the fasting period is over. The women in this study also experienced a 50% increase in their cortisol levels. Cortisol is more commonly referred to as the stress hormone.

Cortisol becomes elevated when we are worn out, nervous, afraid, and/or hungry. It can also cause us to crave sugary, fatty foods to try and feed our body a quick burst of highly available energy. The body craves this quick fix in order to deal with whatever short term situation we are in. This is simply another one of the body's survival mechanisms. As a woman, if you are following intermittent fasting to lose weight, the last thing you want is your cortisol level through the roof, begging you to eat that candy bar or drink a soda. So how can you avoid these hormonal cravings causing you to overeat and desire junk food? Well, instead of going on an extended fast such as 24 to 48 hours, if you will simply narrow your food intake into 8-10 hour feeding windows, you can reap the benefits of intermittent fasting while burning fat and increasing your insulin sensitivity without throwing your hunger hormones for a loop.

Another serious side effect of intermittent fasting unique to the female body is a disrupted menstrual cycle and even a decreased ovary size. A study conducted using female rats found that after two weeks of intermittent fasting, the rat's menstrual cycles ceased completely and their ovaries were severely diminished. This is thought to be yet another survival mechanism in the mammalian body, and sort of makes sense if you think about it. If the female body believes that it is starving, and is trying to use as little energy available as efficiently possible, the last thing that needs to be introduced into this equation is a growing fetus that requires an enormous amount of energy to develop.

If a woman's body believes it is having a hard enough time keeping itself alive, Mother Nature will make some changes, such as bringing ovulation to a halt and shrinking the ovaries. This is to ensure that there will be only one human to keep alive for the time being. While this is a remarkable mechanism of survival that probably served our ancient ancestors well, you are not actually starving, and you most likely do not want to have your reproductive system thrown out of balance. So if you begin intermittent fasting and notice changes in your menstrual cycle and ovulation frequency, what can you do? Dr. Amy Shah, an expert of intermittent fasting protocols and their effects on the female anatomy, recommends what she calls crescendo fasting.

What this entails is that women do not actually fast everyday, but select two to three days out of the week, preferably nonconsecutive days such as Monday, Wednesday, and Friday, and fast the usual 12-16 hours during these days. On the days you are fasting, this method recommends women only engage in physical exercise such a light yoga, while saving any high intensity workouts for non-fasting days. After following this method for 2-3 weeks, women are encouraged to try and add one more fasting day during the week, and monitor their body's reaction. By partaking in crescendo fasting, women are more likely to see the benefits of intermittent fasting without their hormones and reproductive system going into all out panic mode.

While we are on the topic of possible disruptions to the female reproductive system, we will discuss a rather odd side effect that some women may possibly experience from intermittent fasting. The female body contains many unique biological mechanisms that are used specifically to aid in pregnancy and ensure the health of a fetus. Unfortunately, but also incredibly admirable, the female body is designed so that in times of hardship, such as starvation, the fetus will survive no matter the costs to the mother.

When resources and nutrition is running low, a growing fetus can actually cause hormonal changes in the woman's body to reroute vital nutrients to itself. Often when women are following any sort of fasting protocol, when they break the fast they experience severe, insatiable hunger. This is the female body's way of protecting a potential fetus, regardless if there is one or there's not. Because a woman's body is so uniquely designed to develop and nourish a growing baby, it will actually do whatever it takes to maintain an internal environment conducive to a baby's growth, even if there isn't one there!

To mitigate effects such as this one, experts recommend that women go for several trial fasts before diving headfirst into intermittent fasting. This can be done by consuming all food in an 8-hour feeding window maybe once a week, seeing how your body responds to this, and then adding a day if things go smoothly. However if you choose to try out fasting, the key is to be gentle. The last thing you want is to begin an intense fasting regimen and make your body think famine has come and all will be lost if it doesn't protect your growing bundle of joy that isn't actually there. The take home factor is if you choose to begin intermittent fasting, ease into it and the benefits will follow suit.

Another hormonal issue that women need to consider when beginning intermittent fasting, is their estrogen levels. While the male and female bodies both contain estrogen as well as testosterone, we all know that males contain much more testosterone than women, and women more estrogen than men. These hormones work to provide certain physical and emotional aspects that are unique to the different genders.

Estrogen, the primary female sex hormone, can actually make it harder or easier for a woman to stick with any dietary plan, especially intermittent fasting. The different craving levels will change depending on certain periods of the menstrual cycle throughout the month. The reason for this is because the hormone estrogen actually decreases appetite by reducing a woman's sensitivity to feeding cues, causing you to feel hungry less often. At certain periods in the menstrual cycle, such as the per ovulatory phase, food intake is at its lowest. Likewise, during later periods in the menstrual cycle such as the follicular and luteal phases, food intake is actually increased.

But what does this mean for you? Well, assuming that you plan to commit to intermittent fasting as a lifestyle, you are likely to have certain periods of the month when it just seems harder to stick to your feeding window. You may think you are just not exercising enough self-control, or that you are slacking in your commitment to eating healthier, when really you are just the victim of a hormonal fluctuation that's out of your control. While there is no way to stop the fluctuation of estrogen in your body, (none that you want to try anyway) you can mitigate the intense hunger cravings in the same way that we've talked about reducing or preventing other unwanted side effects. Exercise moderation with intermittent fasting, especially when you first begin this lifestyle. As a female, your body is extremely sensitive to hormonal alterations and is likely to respond adversely if you go from your normal eating routine straight into a prolonged fast.

Although this chapter may seem to have portrayed intermittent fasting in a negative light, the hazards that we have discussed are all easily avoidable. As a woman, your body is designed to protect not only you, but even another human life growing inside of you through the body's delicate hormone balance and biological mechanisms. As long as you approach intermittent fasting from a reasonable perspective with this new found awareness, I truly believe that you can experience the many benefits available from this lifestyle, without falling victim to the possible detriments that are out there.

Remember that moderation is key when starting this protocol. The body is extremely intelligent at sensing small changes or fluctuations in your internal and external environments. The body will turn to drastic measures to protect itself and maintain homeostasis. Therefore, when beginning any sort of new diet or exercise program, you should gradually implement the change into your day-to-day life.

You would never attempt to run a marathon without starting a progressive training program. Maybe running a mile every day until that became easy, and then moving on to running halfmarathons, etc. The same logic applies to intermittent fasting. It's not a good idea to go from eating your normal breakfast, lunch, and dinner, then suddenly go 16 hours without eating.

You know when you see those commercials play on television advertising a type of medicine? Then at the end of the ad an unnecessarily fast speaker chimes in to list off about 50 possible side effects listed in the fine print at the bottom of your screen? Although the side effects they mention only occur in a very small percentage of individuals that take the medicine, they still have to inform you of them for your health and safety. This chapter serves that purpose and thoroughly explains any of the female issues that could possibly arrive, so you are aware of them and know how to avoid them.

Although there are some possible health hazards that can occur for women seeking intermittent fasting as a healthy eating habit, this is only the exception to the rule. If you will follow the advice on how to prevent the side effects that we have discussed, you are more than likely to have a pleasant and beneficial experience as you begin this journey. Even ibuprofen has been known to cause everything from diarrhea to shortness of breath in some people, but I doubt that you consider these side effects every time you get a headache! Rest assured that with careful planning and self-awareness, intermittent fasting will help the large majority of women achieve their weight loss and fitness goals.

Chapter 16: Types of Intermittent Fasting

First of all before you get to choose your preferred method of intermittent fasting it's important that you calculate your caloric intake which you will be following throughout your journey. As I have mentioned in previous chapters when you implement intermittent fasting it does make it hard to over eat but it can happen so using this calculation and counting calories will guarantee you succeed.

This is the exact calorie calculation that I used to drop 55 pounds as well as using it with countless of my clients in the past to achieve their body goals. You might think that counting calories is a massive chore and you are not interested in doing so and that's fine, you should still be able to make big strides with your body without doing it, however for those who are interested I suggest you download a calorie counting app of your choice, I use the "my fitness pal" app . The free version is fine and it makes counting calories absolutely effortless.

Woman- your body weight in pounds multiplied by 1012

Eg- for a 147 pound female it would be 147 multiplied by 10 = 1470

Or
147 multiplied by 12 = 1764

So you would be consuming between 1470 and 1764 calories per day

From there you would then break up your calorie intake into your macros of protein, carbs and fats as discussed a few chapters earlier.

Now on to choosing your method of fasting, the most important thing to understand when attempting intermittent fasting is that it should work for you. Everyone's body is different and so intermittent fasting may have different effects on different people. Luckily, people have found many variations of IF that allows people to stick with the program without necessarily hurting their bodies or dying of starvation. If you are new at this and are struggling to find a way to make it work, then this part will be useful to you. Observe the following different ways of intermittent fasting, and pick the one that is most suitable for you.

Alternate-Days Fasting

This is also known as the Up-Day-Down-Day diet. It basically means that you fast one day and then eat the other day. For example, you could fast on Mondays and Wednesdays, then eat normally on the other days. There are many variations to this type of intermittent fasting. One of the most popular ones involves you completely avoiding all solid foods during the fasting days. For others, you are allowed up to 500 calories (making sure that 200 are in the form of protein) during the days that you fast. There is also another variation where you consume water and 500 calories for the first 24 hours then eat as much as you want for the following 24 hours.

The common thing with all of these variations is that on feeding days, people often eat as much and as often as they would like. This type of IF is perfect for people who like routine but also want the freedom to indulge regularly; one day on, then one day off. Studies have shown that alternate fasting is effective for both heart health and weight loss especially in overweight adults.

Daily Window Fasting

This is the most popular way of intermittent fasting because it can be used by almost all types of people. Basically, what this type of fasting means is that you skip meals according to your level of hunger at different times of the day. This is the best type of intermittent fasting for beginners because you will be able to control what time you go hungry and what time you eat. It is easier for everyone because this is how most people actually eat. For example, you could eat breakfast and lunch then skip dinner.

Another popular method is skipping breakfast then start to eat later in the day such as during lunch hours. You can also choose to eat one big meal per day or even observe timeframes of six, three, or one hour depending on your hunger levels. If you are a beginner, the best way to do this is to not eat if you are not really hungry. You can also do a short fast if you travel somewhere and cannot find something good, familiar, or healthy to eat.

Keto Fasting

The keto diet in simple terms is a type of diet where you avoid carbohydrates completely and instead indulge in fatty foods to help maintain metabolism. Keto fasting or fat fasting is a way for breaking a weight loss plateau for people who have already adopted the keto diet and have achieved a state of ketosis. Basically, you will be carrying on with your keto diet and combine it with fasting where you limit your fat intake to specific times of the day. The benefit of this is that the high amount of fats being consumed will help to keep you feeling full and so you will not feel as hungry as you would expect. It also allows you to stay in natural ketosis so that you will not be going back on your diet. However, this type of IF should only be attempted by people who are used to the keto diet already. This is because it limits what you can eat and makes it monotonous and boring. Also, it should not be done long term due to the low-calorie intake combined with scheduled fasting.

It should not be done for more than three to five days at a time in my opinion.

The 5:2 Diet

This is yet another popular type of IF. This type of fasting means that you eat well and normally five days of the week then reduce your calorie intake during the other 2 days of the week. During the fasting days, men consume up to 600 calories and women consume 500 calories. The most common way that people follow the 5:2 diet is by separating their fasting days. This means that rather than eating normally Monday through Friday, a person can eat normally on Sunday to Tuesday, fast on Wednesday, then resume normal diet on Thursday and Friday and then fast again on Saturday. This is just an example as people use different forms. The basic rule is there should be at least one non-fasting day between the two fasting days.

Studies have shown that this type of fasting has resulted in substantial weight loss in overweight people. This diet has also been proven to reduce insulin levels in diabetic people and improve the insulin levels among the people who follow it.

The Warrior Diet

This type of intermittent fasting is perceived to be the most difficult to achieve. It is only attempted by people with a strong will and high level of discipline, hence its name. The warrior diet involves the person eating small amounts of vegetables, fruits, and fat-assimilating proteins such as yogurt every few hours during the day and then eating a very big meal in the last few hours of the night. In other words, you will fast all through the day and feast in the night in a maximum window of four hours only. This type of fasting is best suited for people who have already tried other methods of intermittent fasting and are familiar with it. Supporters of this type of IF claim humans to be natural nocturnal eaters and that through eating at night, the body gains more nutrients in line with its circadian rhythms. However, as stated before, it is not suitable for beginners because it can be challenging to maintain a strict deadline. A big meal close to bedtime is difficult to handle for most people, and there is the risk that you will not get enough nutrients such as fiber. This has adverse effects on the digestive tract in the long run.

Eat Stop Eat

Eat stop eat fasting means fasting for a time of 24 hours once or twice every week. On the days that you are eating, you may decide on three meals every day. As long as you are eating in a responsible manner and keeping their intake in check, then any pattern of meals would be acceptable. Apparently, there is evidence from experts such as Brad Pilon, a weight loss guru that brief regular fasts promote weight loss and the retention of muscle in a better manner than the diets which are there to eliminate particular foods or cut down on the number of calories.

Eat stop eat works in a simplistic manner where the person fasts once or twice on a weekly basis. For example, you may eat normally up to 7 PM on a Saturday and then fast up to 7 PM on Sunday, and then resuming regular eating during that period. If you are not able to make it for the entire 24 hours, then 20 to 24 hours could also work appropriately. For the next few days, you would take in about 2,000 calories every day if you are female or 2,500 if you are a male. It is not advisable for a person to fast on consecutive days as well. After a number of normal eating days, it is possible to embark on a subsequent fast and then go on with the schedule as normal.

During the days when a person is fasting, it is better if them to take in as few calories as possible. The recommendations are for them to only consume sparkling water, diet soda, and coffee. At the time when they break their fast, then it is possible for them to eat anything that they want but this should be done in moderation because overeating can also undo some of the benefits of the fast. You do not have to particularly avoid any particular foods like carbs.

As a matter of fact, a low-carb set diet on the non-fasting days could negatively affect the energy levels. It is better to consume a lot of vegetables, spices, and fruits.

While you are also doing the Eat Stop Eat regimen, you should do some weight training in to help manage and build the muscle rather than cardio or other exercises which are quite exhaustive. It is not necessary for you to exercise during the same days that the fast is taking place though. The guide for Eat Stop Eat regimen recommends that you have a consistent training schedule that goes at three to four times every week with two or four exercises for every body part, six to 15 reps for every set.

Research is currently in support of intermittent fasting as the best mode for weight loss. A review on intermittent calorie restriction which follows a similar schedule to the eat stop eat regimen found it was effective in calorie reduction by a set amount every day leading to weight loss. As such, Eat-Stop-Eat helps dieters retain more lean muscle mass. This approach to intermittent fasting also comes with its own set of health benefits. Apparently fasting on alternate days has been proven to lower the risk of chronic disease in animals though there is a need for more studies to confirm the effects on human beings. Eat stop eat may also be less confusing and straightforward compared to diets in where you have to limit an entire food group like carbs or fat.

Leangains

Leangains was originally coined by Martin Berkhan and is a diet workout that is based on intermittent fasting and lifting huge weights. It is meant to be an approach of body re-composition for losing fat and gaining muscle in the most effective manner. The way it works is 14 hours for women and 16 hours for men, followed by a feeding period of the remaining 8 or 10 hours although there is no reason why women cant fast for 16 hours in our opinion. It works just fine and is totally safe. When the person following this regime is fasting, there no consumption of any calories, although diet soda, black coffee, and sugar-free gum are allowed.

A lot of people see it as one of the more favorable fasts through the night and into the morning period. They may break the fast about six hours after waking up. This is something which can be adapted to the lifestyle of the individual while still maintaining a window where they can eat. In any case, the hormones in the body may be confused and make sticking to the program a bit hard for the person who is doing it.

The food and the time a person eat during the feeding window are dependent on when the exercise takes place. On the days where they exercise, carbs are much more significant compared to fat because you need energy right there and then. On the rest days, the intake of fats should be higher compared to the sugars if there is any intake at all. The intake of protein should be relatively high every day though this is going to vary according to gender, goals, age and the levels of activity. In spite of the particular program, the whole unprocessed foods ought to be the majority of the intake of calories. Though, when there is no time for a meal, then a protein shake or a meal replacement bar would be acceptable.

For many people following the lean gains approach, the advantage is on the number of days the meal frequency would not be relevant. It is possible to eat anything you like within the eight-hour period for feeding. Even so, a lot of people find that dissecting it into three meals is easier to abide by. On the other hand, even though lean gains allows flexibility in when you eat, there are strict specifications on the composition of the diet especially when it comes to when you are working out. The nutrition plan and scheduling meals perfectly around workouts would make the program harder to adhere to. If you are interested in focusing purely on the 16/8 method we have a book on Amazon that you might be interested in called Intermittent Fasting 16/8, just search for Rebekah Addams and it should come up

Fat Loss Forever

This approach toward intermittent fasting takes some of the better parts from the warrior diet, eat stop eat, and lean gains, and then combines it into one plan. It is also possible to get one cheat day every week which is followed by a 36-hour fast. After this, then the remainder of the seven-day cycle would be split between the different fasting type protocols. There are some who have suggested having the longest fasts take place on the days when they are the busiest as this allows them to be focused on being more productive than anything else. This plan also considers training programs such as free weights and bodyweight in order to assist the person in being able to reach the maximum amount of fat loss in the simplest manner.

The advantage when it comes to the fat loss forever approach is while everyone is technically fasting each day, during the time that you are not working, it is not structured and this approach allows for just that. There is a seven-day schedule so that the body can get used to the structured timetable in order for it to get the most from the periods. Similarly, there is a full cheat day at the end of it which you can work towards in order to reward yourself for being so diligent during the week. Now, the trouble is if you have problems handling the cheat days in a reasonable and healthy way, then the method is not going to work out for you. At the same time, because the plan is particular and the feeding and fasting schedule is dependent from day to day, the method can be confusing to follow.

Though, the plan does come with a calendar with a schedule to fast and exercise every day.

Up Day Down Day

This is an easy approach as the practitioner eats very little the first day and then eats normally the next. When it comes to the low-calorie days that would be a fraction of the normal calorie intake, the figure of 2,000 would be downgraded to about 500 calories for that day. In order to make the down days that much easier for you to comply, it is recommended to opt for meal replacement type shakes for the protein. These are strengthened with the essential nutrients and you are able to sip them throughout the entire day as opposed to splitting them into small meals.

The thing is meal replacement shakes only ought to be done during the first two weeks of this diet approach. After this, it would be advisable for you to eat real food during the down days. The next day should be a normal day where you eat the way you would normally but with healthy portions of everything. It may be advisable as well for you to keep any workout schedules slim on these days or save the exercise sessions for the days you do normal calorie intake.

The great thing with the up-day down-day approach is that it is all about the loss of weight so if you just want to reduce your overall weight and get a little fit, then this would be the approach to take. On average, people who cut calories by 20 to 35 percent tend to see losses of about two and a half pounds every week. Now, though the approach is very easy to understand and follow, it may be very tempting for the people doing it to give in to temptation on the normal or up days and decide to binge eat. The best way for you to stay on track would be planning the meals ahead of time wherever possible so that there is no chance of getting caught off guard. It needs a higher level of discipline to stay on point especially during the down days but also on the up days. This means maybe setting aside an hour or 2 per week as your meal prep time so that you have all of your food readily available when you need it.

My personal approach

While the all of these methods are well known in regard to integrating periods of fasting to the eating schedule, there are a number of philosophies that are based according to meal timing. For the ones that prefer more fluid and less rigid methods, there would be the concept of eating more intuitively. This would be when hunger is there and when the body requests nutrients. Some claim this can also lead to overeating or over-consuming of the calories since the body's hunger-induced choices can either be related to calories or cravings that are essentially harmful to the person. Of course, fasting, regardless of the approach, is not for everyone because it requires some type of discipline in order for whoever is following it to be successful. It does not matter which type you go for — there is no easy option. Of course, there are some that are more extreme than others, but the fact is that all types need intense investment and commitment from the person involved.

I don't follow a specific method, all I do is simply aim to fast a minimum of 4-6 hours upon waking up in the morning. If you include my sleep time then a lot of times that will work out very similar to the 16/8 method although there are plenty of times when my fasting time works out to be less than 16 hours as well as sometimes being more. I don't stick to a certain style therefor I don't beat myself up if I cant follow things to a tee on any given day.

The only rules I do stick with is my calorie count. I would out my maintenance level caloric intake and I increase that number slightly if I am trying to put on some lean muscle or use the calculations that I explained earlier in this chapter if I am trying to burn fat. I keep my protein intake high following the bodyweight in pounds multiplied by 0.82 calculation that I mentioned in a previous chapter and as far as my fats and carbs go I just eat a moderate amount of both.

It doesn't have to be over complicated, I don't follow any type of diet within the intermittent fasting protocol, I eat "normal" and "real" foods so long as you get a few serves of fruit and vegetables every day you will be healthy on the inside and out. Regardless what many health professionals and fitness experts tell you, you don't need to eat boring chicken breast, brown rice and broccoli 6 times a day to get and stay in shape.

Chapter 17 Tips for Success

While each type of intermittent fasting is beneficial in its way, they can also each be very complicated and confusing to stick within both the long and the short term if you don't tackle them with the right mindset. The suggestions found in the following pages can make the process much more comfortable, however, so it is recommended that you give them a try before throwing in the towel and going back to your old unhealthy or lazy eating habits.

Stay true to yourself: While intermittent fasting can indeed provide you with a variety of healthy lifestyle changes, it doesn't mean it is going to be the right choice for everyone. While you should be able to make it through some fasts without slipping, once you have done so you are going to want to consider how difficult that period was for you. You will also need to think what your natural habits are like when it comes to eating and what your overall relationship with food is like in general. It is essential to keep in mind that intermittent fasting is not so much a diet as it is a lifestyle which means you should focus on long term success and not think about it as a short-term solution like you would most diets.

This long-term commitment is why you are going to want to seriously ask yourself if you are going to be able to commit to fasting regularly in the long term, if not with the first type of intermittent fasting that you try then possibly the second or the third. If you have a long way to go when it comes to meeting your weight loss goals, then you may want to start with something milder than intermittent fasting and instead work up to it once you have gotten into the habit of eating healthy first. Starting off with a style of eating that has an extreme learning curve can lead to early failure that can affect you mentally and make you less likely to try again.

Be aware of what your body is trying to tell you: While adjusting to intermittent fasting will almost always come with some side effects, it is important to remember that these are supposed to fade in time which means you are going to want to remain in touch with your body to ensure you don't end up hurting yourself in the process. If you find yourself experiencing more prolonged or more severe symptoms, it is essential to stop immediately instead of powering through. Maintaining your overall health is critical when it comes to maximizing the results from intermittent fasting, and you can't do that if your body is reacting negatively to the process. Listen to the things your body is telling you and never try to push yourself past your limits, if you do, you could find yourself passing out from hunger, or worse.

Don't expect too much, too soon: It is essential to keep in mind that initially, when you switch to an intermittent fasting plan you are likely not going to lose weight for the first week or so as your body reacts to the change. From there, you may experience a period of higher than normal weight loss for a time. However this will not last, and as your body fully adapts to the change, you will likely start to see a weight loss of about 1 pound per week, which is the average amount of healthy weight loss recommended by experts.

Additionally, you are going to need to keep in mind that everyone hits weight loss plateaus, regardless of how strictly they are following their chosen weight loss plan. This is an unavoidable part of losing weight and if you take that as an excuse to mix things up with a new type of intermittent fasting or to naturally fall off the wagon you are going to be doing yourself a great disservice. Changing horses midstream is only going to confuse your body without making you lose weight any faster and falling off the wagon has never done anyone any right regardless of the specifics of the situation. Stay the course, and you will be back on track before you know it. An idea may be to bring your daily calories up for 3 or 4 weeks. I would suggest around 300 calories for a female and around 500 calories for a male, you shouldn't put on any weight during this time but if you do, don't panic. This raise in calories will shock your body and snap it back out of the plateau and when you return to your normal calorie intake you should continue to lose weight.

Don't let yourself make excuses: While it is essential not to get started on a new intermittent fasting plan when your schedule is hectic, or you have extra stress or anxiety on your plate, it is also important to not keep putting it off every time something new comes up. Life is always going to be busy, that is why one of the benefits of intermittent fasting is having more time each fasting day. At some point, the reasons you have for putting it off are merely going to be excused to avoid getting started. Be frank with yourself and understand that there is always going to be something standing in your way from making positive life changes. You just need to power through it if you ever hope to see real success.

At some point, all you can do is say enough is enough and get down to business. After all, the only person that can motivate you to stick with a healthy intermittent fasting diet plan in the long term is you. This is why it is so important not to let yourself down. If you truly commit to finding personal success when it comes to your weight loss goals, then there should be nothing that can stop you. It is as simple as that.

Chapter 18: Exercise & Intermittent Fasting

One common question people have when doing intermittent fasting is whether or not it is safe and healthy to exercise either aerobically or anaerobically while they are "running on empty" so to speak. If done correctly, the combination can help you burn lots of your body's fat reserves quickly. Maintaining some exercise routine is vital for your mental and physical health – that's a given. So, in fact, exercising and running in a fasted state is a great way to become fat adapted and improve your mental state of mind at the same time.

You've already heard the adage, 80% diet, 20% exercise – to combine dieting with training. This is true! Imagine if we could make our body burn more fat for fuel while at rest, and they also burn fat more efficiently during exercise. Most of us have around 40,000 calories of fat in our bodies at any given time and around 1,200 calories of muscle glycogen or sugar. Imagine how far or how much we could exercise if we had access to that 40,000calorie fuel tank. That's 33 times the amount of energy fuel! So, perhaps next time you run out of energy in the middle of an exercise routine, you will wish your body was in fat-burning mode instead of calorie-burning mode.

The first step to burning more fat during exercise is: you need to have what's called an "aerobic base." The way to build this base is thru aerobic heart rate training, which will raise what is known as your "aerobic capacity." Aerobic capacity is defined as the maximal amount of oxygen in milliliters (ml) that an athlete utilizes in one minute, per kilogram of body weight. In layman's terms, the higher the "aerobic base" or "capacity," the more body-work you can do in one minute. The best method I have found for heart rate training is Phil Maffetone's "MAF" training.

I have included a link to his paper on heart rate training here. What does this mean for exercise? Technically, by having a higher aerobic base, we boost the size and strength of our heart, the concentration of hemoglobin in our blood, the density of our capillaries, and the number of mitochondria in our muscles. The benefits expand beyond the scope of this book, but mostly by developing an aerobic base, we become healthier inside and out.

What this means for intermittent fasting is that when you are training in a fasted state, your body becomes superbly efficient at burning fat for fuel. From an aerobic aspect your body can more efficiently utilize oxygen and this, in turn, makes you more productive at exercise aerobically or anaerobically. You must first develop your aerobic base to enhance anaerobic exercise. If you wanted to learn more on this subject you can check Phil Maffetone's website for more details.

If you are looking to add muscle, fasting can help by increasing the production of certain hormones in your body. Other than weight training and getting the proper amount of sleep regularly, fasting has proven to be one of the most effective methods of increasing human growth hormone as I spoke about earlier in this book." Studies have also suggested that fasting in combination with regular exercise can increase the levels of testosterone in men and women, which is another hormone that can decrease body fat and increase muscle mass. Here are my recommendations for adding muscle:

- Don't push yourself too hard. If you are doing "cardio" exercise, as a test, make sure you can carry on a conversation at the same time; otherwise, you may be pushing yourself too hard. When you are doing the exercise slowly, but for a long time, that's when your body is becoming more "fat adapted." That's when it is going into a ketogenic state. Listen always to your body, and stop if you start to feel dizzy or lightheaded.

- The 16/8 method, in particular, recommends scheduling your meals for when you plan to finish doing any moderate-to-intense exercise. Plan your high-intensity workouts for around a time when you are getting ready to break your fast so that you can eat soon after that. Adequately scheduled, if your workout is very intense, you can follow it with a carbohydrate-rich snack.

- If you are lifting weights, make sure you are getting adequate protein or supplementing with adequate BCAAs. "Feast" on meals that are high in protein. Eating protein on a regular basis is vital for muscle growth.

- When planning your meals with workouts in mind, try combining fast-acting simple carbohydrates with a protein that will serve to stabilize your blood sugar after your workout. A banana and some peanut butter is a good example.

Conclusion

Thanks for making it through to the end of *Intermittent Fasting for Women*. Let's hope it was informative and able to provide you with all of the tools you need to achieve your goals — whatever they may be.

The next step is to evaluate your eating options for a period of the last few years and honestly consider your relationship with food. The intermittent fasting schedule is there to change the strategy of how you relate to food. Instead of food dictating what and when you eat, you regain this power and put an end to harmful addictions that may be causing health problems in your life.

As indicated in the text, intermittent fasting assists with a variety of issues from cancer and diabetes to epilepsy. It even helps you live longer and improves brain activity. Who would have thought that your relationship with food can dictate the length of your life or the quality of it. Society passes on ideas backed by capitalist organizations about food and this becomes adopted by people who are not mindful about the way their bodies work. The body was not meant to be endlessly punished up to the point of disease and even death. You could say this is a way for you to break free from the hold food has on you so that you can become a better and more productive person. After all, this is a lifestyle guide through which you can better yours and the lives of others.

Hopefully, by following the example you set, others may also be saved from a wasteful lifestyle. If you need help on the intermittent diet, you can consider one of the diet types as indicated towards the end of the book. Work with the one that suits you the best or caters to your unique schedule as you have seen my personal plan is not as strict as many of the other types of intermittent fasting as that suits my situation. You know what type of person you are, your strengths and weaknesses, be honest with yourself and chose the format of intermittent fasting that's going to be the easiest for you to stick with. Become a leader in health and positive body image to inspire others who do not know about the diet and are looking for ways to better their eating patterns.

Also another reminder to look up our free accountability group on facebook called **Intermittent Fasting, Fuel the Brain, Lose the Fat** and to claim your Intermittent Fasting Cheat Sheet at **www.thefastingfacts.com.**

Finally, if you found this book useful in any way, a review on Amazon is always appreciated!

!

References

Brown, Paige. (2018). Eat, Fast and Refeed Mindfully: Mindful Eating May Boost Metabolic Health. Retrieved from https://medium.com/lifeomic/eat-fast-and-refeed-mindfullymindful-eating-may-boost-metabolic-health-a87779546f46

O'Donnell, Mike. (2018). Break Bad Eating Habits with Intermittent Fasting. retrieved from http://www.theiflife.com/break-bad-eating-habits

Rush, Raymond. (2018). Intermittent Fasting and Diabetes: A Safe Eating Plan for People with Type 2? Retrieved from https://www.ontrackdiabetes.com/live-well/eatwell/intermittent-fasting-diabetes-safe-eating-plan-peopletype-2

Henriques, Carolina. (2016). Fasting May Help to Prevent Seizures by Calming Nervous System, Early Study Suggests. Retrieved from https://epilepsynewstoday.com/2016/12/16/fasting-mayreduce-epileptic-seizures-by-calming-nervous-system

Omodei D, Fontana L (2011) Calorie restriction and prevention of age-associated chronic disease. FEBS Lett585:1537-1542.

Salcido, Brady. (2017). 6 Surprising Brain Power Benefits of Intermittent Fasting. retrieved from https://medium.com/@drbradysalcido/6-surprising-brainpower-benefits-of-intermittent-fasting-49ad1bc39e04

Revelant, Judy. (2017). Is Intermittent Fasting Safe for People with Diabetes? Retrieved from https://www.everydayhealth.com/type-2-

diabetes/diet/intermittent-fasting-safe-people-with-diabetes

Cathy, Leman. (2018). Could Intermittent Fasting Be the Answer to Reducing Breast Cancer Recurrence Risk? Retrieved from http://dammadaboutbreastcancer.com/dont-read-yourenighttime-eater

Made in the USA
Monee, IL
12 February 2021